S0-AFW-083

CT Urography

An Atlas

CT Urography
An Atlas

Stuart G. Silverman, MD
Professor of Radiology
Harvard Medical School
Director, Abdominal Imaging and Intervention
Director, CT Scan
Director, Cross-sectional Interventional Service
Department of Radiology
Brigham and Women's Hospital
Boston, Massachusetts

Richard H. Cohan, MD
Professor of Radiology
University of Michigan
Associate Chair for Education
Associate Residency Training Program Director
Department of Radiology
University of Michigan Hospital
Ann Arbor, Michigan

Wolters Kluwer | Lippincott Williams & Wilkins
Health

Acquisitions Editor: Lisa McAllister
Managing Editor: Kerry Barrett
Developmental Editor: Franny Murphy
Project Manager: Jennifer Harper
Manufacturing Coordinator: Kathleen Brown
Marketing Manager: Angela Panetta
Creative Director: Doug Smock
Production Services: GGS Book Services
Printer: Walsworth Publishing Company

© 2007 by LIPPINCOTT WILLIAMS & WILKINS, a Wolters Kluwer business
530 Walnut Street
Philadelphia, PA 19106 USA
LWW.com

All rights reserved. This book is protected by copyright. No part of this book may be reproduced in any form or by any means, including photocopying, or utilized by any information storage and retrieval system without written permission from the copyright owner, except for brief quotations embodied in critical articles and reviews. Materials appearing in this book prepared by individuals as part of their official duties as U.S. government employees are not covered by the above-mentioned copyright.

Printed in the USA

Library of Congress Cataloging-in-Publication Data
CT urography : an atlas / [edited by] Stuart G. Silverman, Richard H.
   Cohan.
     p. ; cm.
   ISBN-13: 978-0-7817-8754-3
   ISBN-10: 0-7817-8754-8
   1. Genitourinary organs—Radiography—Atlases. 2. Tomography—Atlases.
3. Genitourinary organs—Diseases—Diagnosis—Atlases. I. Silverman, Stuart G.
II. Cohan, Richard H.
   [DNLM: 1. Urography—methods—Atlases. 2. Urography—methods—Case Reports.
3. Tomography, X-Ray Computed—Atlases. 4. Tomography, X-Ray Computed—
Case Reports.   WJ 17 C959 2007]
RC874.U76 2007
616.6'0757—dc22   2006025299

Care has been taken to confirm the accuracy of the information presented and to describe generally accepted practices. However, the authors, editors, and publisher are not responsible for errors or omissions or for any consequences from application of the information in this book and make no warranty, expressed or implied, with respect to the currency, completeness, or accuracy of the contents of the publication. Application of this information in a particular situation remains the professional responsibility of the practitioner.

The authors, editors, and publisher have exerted every effort to ensure that drug selection and dosage set forth in this text are in accordance with current recommendations and practice at the time of publication. However, in view of ongoing research, changes in government regulations, and the constant flow of information relating to drug therapy and drug reactions, the reader is urged to check the package insert for each drug for any change in indications and dosage and for added warnings and precautions. This is particularly important when the recommended agent is a new or infrequently employed drug.

Some drugs and medical devices presented in this publication have Food and Drug Administration (FDA) clearance for limited use in restricted research settings. It is the responsibility of the health care provider to ascertain the FDA status of each drug or device planned for use in their clinical practice.

To purchase additional copies of this book, call our customer service department at (800) 638-3030 or fax orders to (301) 223-2320. International customers should call (301) 223-2300.

Visit Lippincott Williams & Wilkins on the Internet: at LWW.com. Lippincott Williams & Wilkins customer service representatives are available from 8:30 am to 6pm, EST.

10 9 8 7 6 5 4 3 2 1

DEDICATION

To my parents, Alan and Estelle Silverman, for their wisdom, support, and life-long love, and to my loving wife, Tricia, and our proudest and most joyous achievements, Alex, Stacy, and Michael.

STUART G. SILVERMAN, MD

To my parents, Julian and Greta Cohan, for their kindness, support, and love through all these many years. Also to my wife, Nina, for her love, perseverance, and tolerance of me being me, and to our four almost all grown-up children, Adam, Alex, Charlie, and Rebeka.

RICHARD H. COHAN, MD

CONTRIBUTORS

Elaine M. Caoili, MD
Associate Professor of Radiology
University of Michigan
Department of Radiology
University of Michigan Hospital
Ann Arbor, Michigan

Richard H. Cohan, MD
Professor of Radiology
University of Michigan
Associate Chair for Education
Associate Residency Training Program Director
Department of Radiology
University of Michigan Hospital
Ann Arbor, Michigan

Nigel Cowan, MD, FRCP, FRCR
Honorable Senior Lecturer
Department of Radiology
Oxford, University
Consultant Radiologist
Department of Radiology
The Churchill Hospital
Oxford, United Kingdom

N. Reed Dunnick, MD
Fred Jenner Hodges Professor of Radiology
University of Michigan
Chairman
Department of Radiology
University of Michigan Hospital
Ann Arbor, Michigan

Elliot K. Fishman, MD
Professor of Radiology and Oncology
Director, Diagnostic Imaging and Body CT
The Russell H. Morgan Department of
    Radiology and Radiological Science
Johns Hopkins Hospital
Baltimore, Maryland

Susan Hilton, MD
Clinical Professor
Department of Radiology
University of Pennsylvania Medical School
Co-Chief, CT Section
Department of Radiology
Hospital of the University of Pennsylvania
Philadelphia, Pennsylvania

Satomi Kawamoto, MD
Assistant Professor
Department of Radiology
Johns Hopkins Medical Institutions
Johns Hopkins Outpatient Center
Baltimore, Maryland

Sameh K. Morcos, MD, FRCS, FRCR
Professor of Diagnostic Imaging
University of Sheffield
Consultant Radiologist
Department of Diagnostic Imaging
Northern General Hospital
Sheffield, United Kingdom

Richard D. Nawfel, MS
Associate Physicist
Harvard Medical School
Medical Physicist
Department of Radiology
Brigham and Women's Hospital
Boston, Massachusetts

Michael P. O'Leary, MD
Associate Professor
Harvard Medical School
Department of Urology
Brigham and Women's Hospital
Boston, Massachusetts

Joseph P. Silletti, MD
Resident in Urology
Harvard Longwood Program
    in Urology
Harvard Medical School
Department of Urology
Brigham and Women's Hospital
Boston, Massachusetts

Stuart G. Silverman, MD
Professor of Radiology
Harvard Medical School
Director, Abdominal Imaging and Intervention
Director, CT Scan
Director, Cross-sectional Interventional Service
Department of Radiology
Brigham and Women's Hospital
Boston, Massachusetts

Terri J. Vrtiska, MD
Assistant Professor of Radiology
Mayo Clinic College of Medicine
Consultant
Department of Radiology
Mayo Clinic
Rochester, Minnesota

Jonathon M. Willatt, MD
Lecturer II
University of Michigan
Department of Radiology
University of Michigan Hospital
Ann Arbor, Michigan

Lisa M. Zorn, MD
Clinical Fellow in Radiology
Department of Radiology
Harvard Medical School
Resident
Department of Radiology
Brigham and Women's Hospital
Boston, Massachusetts

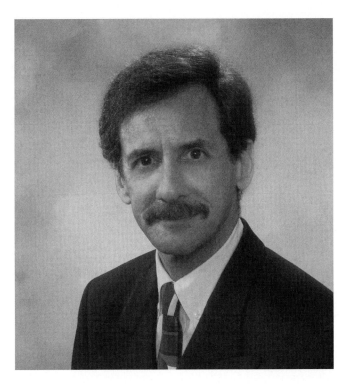 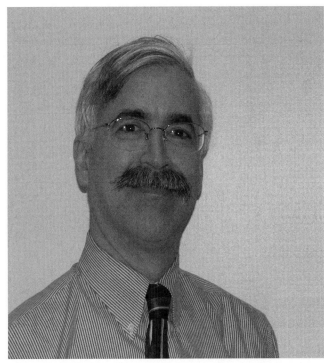

Perhaps one definition of a sentinel event in a procedure-based medical specialty such as radiology would be when one procedure is replaced by a new one. Such has occurred in the field of uroradiology. Intravenous urography, commonly known as the "IVP" and performed since 1929 for a variety of disorders of the urinary tract, has been almost completely replaced by CT urography. In some hospitals and imaging centers, excretory urography suites have been converted for other purposes, and the once standard urinary tract imaging test has all but vanished.

How did this happen? One by one, the indications for intravenous urography have diminished; CT urography is now the test of choice for most anatomic disorders of the kidneys, ureters, and bladder. Innumerable scientific articles in the radiology literature have demonstrated the superiority of CT for evaluating patients with urinary complaints compared not only to intravenous urography but also to ultrasound and MRI. CT has been used for many years to image the urinary tract for renal masses, trauma, infection, stones, and so on. Many of these problems were solved using CT as a result of advances in CT technology. For example, the advent of spiral (helical) CT in the early 1990s allowed

us to obtain a volumetric acquisition of the abdominal cavity such that small stones could be imaged with CT. Just as important, the introduction of multidetector CT allowed us to obtain volumetric images with spatial resolution that rivals conventional radiography. This was the final technological hurdle needed to image the urothelium. As a result, CT urography, an examination that consists of CT scans obtained both before and after the administration of intravenous contrast material, now serves as a fast, single, comprehensive examination of the urinary tract. Several articles in the literature have shown that CT urography can provide images that are markedly better than intravenous urography. Although additional research needs to be done to demonstrate its test characteristics, data show that CT urography is sensitive and specific for detecting and characterizing many anatomic urologic disorders.

This exciting and revolutionary development called for a new textbook in uroradiology. As uroradiologists, we thought the time was right for a book that explained how, when, and why CT urography should be used and, in particular, how to interpret the spectacular images that result. We assembled a short list of many world experts who have conducted much of the research in CT urography to contribute to the book. We chose an atlas format to placate the medical student, resident, fellow, and busy practitioner who are interested in a concise summary of the field. The atlas is buttressed by three textbook-like chapters that focus on the key issues: indications, technique, and radiation exposure. The atlas chapters are then presented in a case format and can be read as unknowns with self-testing. The discussions that follow each case are intended to provide the reader with basic knowledge of the presented entity and how CT urography was used to diagnose it.

CT Urography: An Atlas is not intended to be a comprehensive textbook in uroradiology but, rather, one that reviews the common entities diagnosed with CT urography. Because CT has become one of, if not the most useful imaging examination of the urinary tract, a book that concentrates on urinary tract CT in some respects is long overdue. We are at the precipice of a new era in uroradiology, and with this book, we hope to help radiologists, urologists, nephrologists, and anyone else interested in imaging of the urinary tract embrace this powerful, new technique.

STUART G. SILVERMAN, MD
RICHARD H. COHAN, MD

FOREWORD

The pace of change in radiology, both as a diagnostic tool and as image-guided therapy, has been dramatic. Not only have our imaging modalities become more robust, but improvements in computer technology now enable vast quantities of information to be processed in seconds. These improvements in modalities are most evident in computed tomography.

Uroradiology has benefited from these improvements as much or more than any other subspecialty in radiology. Conventional imaging techniques, such as excretory urography, have been almost completely replaced with CT. Although the superior spatial resolution of radiography as compared with CT would suggest that conventional techniques would still be needed to detect small urothelial lesions, such as transitional cell carcinomas, CT urography is proving to be superior. The improved density differentiation, and the ability to display these CT images in many different projections using different algorithms have enabled CT to define lesions that could not be detected with conventional imaging techniques.

Drs. Silverman and Cohan have been at the leading edge of CT urography. As is often the case in science, investigations from their two independent laboratories have yielded the same conclusion — CT urography is rapidly replacing conventional uroradiological imaging.

Many challenges remain. We must continue to provide exquisite diagnostic imaging while reducing the radiation dose to the patient; refinement in appropriate use of this imaging technology is essential; a better method for analyzing the enormous data sets generated by these examinations is needed; and, finally, there is a generation of radiologists who must be educated in the indications, techniques, and interpretation of these examinations.

Drs. Silverman and Cohan have assembled an international faculty to compile this atlas of CT urography. These authors constitute a "who's who" in the field. The images are multiple and superb. The text is both authoritative and concise. The atlas format will allow students and experienced radiologists alike to learn in a setting that mimics the clinical environment. I am confident this textbook will become an essential addition to all radiology libraries.

N. REED DUNNICK, MD

SPECIAL THANKS

We are forever grateful to the many contributors, listed as authors of the chapters that follow, for their time and expertise in writing portions of this book. They are all busy academicians, and they all graciously agreed to add chapter writing to their full schedules. Because CT urography is a relatively new technique, some chapters needed to be supplemented with "borrowed cases." These cases are specified as such in each chapter, but a special thanks is also warranted here. As with any endeavor that is comparable in magnitude to authoring a book, there are people, other than the listed contributors, who deserve recognition beyond what is in these printed pages. Of course, this book could not have been completed without the efforts of our colleague, Elaine Caoili, who contributed extensively to three chapters in this text. In addition to coauthoring a chapter, Lisa Zorn, while coping with the rigors of radiology residency at the Brigham, donated her time in helping round out some other chapters. Kirsti Dean, while visiting the Abdominal Section from her home in Finland, ably helped build an image library of Brigham CT urography case material from which many of the images were chosen for this book. Koenraad Mortele (while working on a book of his own) was helpful in comparing notes and offering advice on how to format images electronically (for the same publisher). Donna Vega, Dr. Silverman's assistant, lent a helping hand in typing the revisions of many of the chapters and helped with the coordination and communication needed to orchestrate a multiauthored book. Linda Hart, Dr. Cohan's assistant, also contributed mightily to the compilation of many chapters in the book. Heartfelt appreciation is extended to Jim Ellis, whose morale and emotional support could not be valued more highly. Finally, a special thanks is due Lisa McAllister, Kerry Barrett, and the rest of the staff at Lippincott Williams & Wilkins. They believed in the concept of the book and were helpful every step of the way, including their efforts to have the book compiled and released in a very short period of time. They, too, realized the potential of CT urography and the impact that this new and exciting technique is having on the field of uroradiology.

STUART G. SILVERMAN, MD
RICHARD H. COHAN, MD

TABLE OF CONTENTS

CHAPTER NINE URETERS 172
Nigel Cowan

CHAPTER TEN CT UROGRAPHY OF THE BLADDER 209
Richard H. Cohan, Elaine M. Caoili, Jonathon M. Willatt

CHAPTER ELEVEN   CT UROGRAPHY
PITFALLS AND ARTIFACTS   252
Richard H. Cohan, Elaine M. Caoili

CT Urography
An Atlas

CHAPTER ONE

OVERVIEW OF IMAGING OF THE URINARY TRACT AND THE ROLE OF CT UROGRAPHY

JOSEPH P. SILLETTI, MD

MICHAEL P. O'LEARY, MD

From calculus disease to hematuria, imaging has been of great importance in the diagnosis of many diseases of the urinary tract. Advances in imaging technology have changed the practice of uroradiology significantly. CT urography represents one of the most advanced developments in imaging the urinary tract to date. This chapter describes a brief history of uroradiology and focuses on current indications for CT urography. Other imaging modalities are compared, and the role of CT urography in the management of urinary tract disease is discussed.

HISTORY

Early uroradiology techniques were based on the abdominal plain film and were, for the most part, performed for the evaluation of calculus disease (1). Subsequently, retrograde pyelography was developed, and it was first performed with the injection of contrast material directly into the ureters from a cystoscopic approach utilizing colloidal silver, air, carbon dioxide, and other compounds. Retrograde pyelography represented the first imaging study in which contrast material was used to depict anatomy and structural abnormalities.

In 1930, Moses Swick (2), a urologist, developed the first safe intravenous contrast material, Uroselectan, a single iodine atom connected to a pyridine ring. This innovation led to the development of intravenous urography (IVU). With further advancements in the composition of iodinated contrast material in the 1950s and 1960s, the modern intravenous urogram evolved (3). Initially, linear tomography of the kidneys or nephrotomography was added if a renal parenchymal lesion was suspected, and arteriography was performed when the mass was suspicious. In 1974, Bosniak (4) showed that nephrotomography increased the detection of renal masses compared to IVU alone, leading to increased use of this technique. In the late 1970s, ultrasound replaced arteriography as the adjunctive imaging modality of choice for renal masses detected with IVU. Ultrasound, even in its earliest form, was capable of differentiating solid from cystic renal lesions without ionizing radiation or contrast material. In the 1980s and 1990s, CT quickly emerged as a powerful tool in the diagnosis of many diseases of the urinary tract, including renal masses. CT also outperformed other imaging modalities in the diagnosis of renal infection, trauma, and calculi. However, IVU was still needed to image the urothelium. In the late 1990s, MRI became an important modality in the diagnosis of urologic disease, especially in patients with renal insufficiency and in patients with an allergy to iodinated contrast media. Finally, with the advent of multidetector CT, CT became capable of producing a large number of thin section images in a short period of time. As a result, the spatial, temporal, and contrast resolution became sufficient to image the urothelium. Thus, CT could be used to evaluate all major anatomic segments of the urinary tract. Protocols were developed that provided IVU-like images of the urinary tract, referred to as CT urography, and included CT scans of the abdomen and pelvis both before and after the administration of IV contrast material.

INDICATIONS FOR UPPER TRACT IMAGING

CT urography is useful in patients with hematuria. Since hematuria has many causes, a thorough evaluation of both the upper and lower tracts is needed to diagnose malignancy, infection, and other causes of hematuria. CT urography may be used to detect renal masses, urothelial tumors, and the sequelae of complicated infection. CT urography is also useful in the setting of trauma and in the identification and classification of congenital anomalies. An additional important use of CT is in the evaluation of patients with flank pain, in whom unenhanced CT scans are sufficient in most cases. Use of CT or CT urography in evaluating patients with all of the previously mentioned conditions is addressed in the following sections.

Flank Pain Flank pain often requires imaging to discern its etiology. In healthy, young individuals, unilateral flank pain that radiates to the ipsilateral groin is most likely caused by ureterolithiasis. However, in patients with right-sided flank pain or pain radiating to the right lower quadrant, other abdominal pathology, such as appendicitis or ovarian torsion, should also be considered. Therefore, imaging is often needed to diagnose the cause of flank pain. Unenhanced CT has supplanted IVU as the initial test of choice to evaluate patients with flank pain. CT is a faster, more informative, and highly sensitive test that carries no risk of adverse reactions associated with intravenous contrast material (5). In addition, CT can be used to determine a stone's size and position in the ureter, which may facilitate treatment planning.

Nonradiating unilateral flank pain may be a sign of other urinary tract pathology, including renal cell carcinoma. The classic triad of flank pain, palpable mass, and hematuria is uncommon, occurring in only 1% of patients with renal cell carcinoma (6). Indeed, most renal cell carcinomas are discovered incidentally during abdominal imaging performed for nonrenal complaints. Flank pain may also be due to urinary obstruction, typically noted on imaging as hydronephrosis; the discomfort is thought to be due to stretching of the renal capsule. Unilateral hydronephrosis may be secondary to intrinsic or extrinsic causes anywhere along the course of the ureter from the ureteropelvic junction (UPJ) to the ureterovesical junction. Patients with UPJ obstruction present with hydronephrosis in the absence of hydroureter. Most cases of congenital UPJ obstruction are caused by an atonic segment of ureter at the level of the UPJ (noted histologically as an alteration of circular muscle fibers and collagen fibers) (7) or extrinsic compression by a crossing lower pole vessel (8). Congenital UPJ obstruction may be repaired using open surgical or endoscopic approaches.

Congenital abnormalities are less common in adults than children, but they are still important causes of unilateral flank pain and hydronephrosis. Retrocaval and circumcaval ureters may lead to unilateral flank pain (9). Also, the presence of a congenitally duplicated system may have elements of obstruction, as seen in patients with ureteroceles, ectopic ureters, or vesicoureteral reflux (10).

Other common intrinsic causes of unilateral flank pain and hydronephrosis include benign ureteral strictures, typically due to calculus disease, and tumors, the most common of which is transitional cell carcinoma (TSS). Other causes of ureteral strictures include prior pelvic or retroperitoneal surgery, radiation therapy, previous ureteral instrumentation, and trauma.

Extrinsic causes of hydronephrosis are common. Retroperitoneal and pelvic masses, whether benign or malignant, may obstruct the ureter (11). In addition, a number of extrinsic inflammatory causes may lead to ureteral strictures, including primary retroperitoneal fibrosis (12), inflammatory abdominal aortic and iliac aneurysms (13), and diverticulitis (14).

When assessing patients with flank pain, unenhanced CT may be sufficient in diagnosing calculus disease. However, when flank pain is unexplained, or when hydronephrosis is identified and also unexplained, imaging of the entire upper tract is recommended. IVU and retrograde pyelography may both be used to evaluate the ureter for intrinsic causes, but in general, these tests provide a paucity of information regarding extrinsic causes and abnormalities of extraurinary abdominal organs. CT urography can be used to evaluate the entire urinary tract for both intrinsic and extrinsic causes of obstruction and flank pain, and since the whole abdomen and pelvis are imaged, all abdominal and pelvic organs may also be evaluated.

Urinary Tract Infection Infections of the urinary tract are common and usually self-limited. Almost all cases of cystitis are diagnosed on the basis of signs and symptoms alone, treated quickly, and require no imaging. Pyelonephritis, although more serious, is often diagnosed without imaging; however, in some cases, imaging may be needed to confirm the diagnosis. CT urography may be performed to evaluate for a renal or perirenal abscess, emphysematous pyelonephritis, or pyonephrosis in patients with a urinary tract infection who do not respond appropriately to antibiotic therapy. Emphysematous pyelonephritis is an acute necrotizing infection of the renal parenchyma (15). Pyonephrosis (16) is an infection that involves the collecting system usually in the setting of obstructing calculi. Patients with pyonephrosis complain of acute unilateral flank pain, high fever, and, occasionally, nausea and vomiting. These patients are acutely ill and may be septic at presentation.

In patients with chronic fevers, recurrent urinary tract infections, vague flank discomfort, and malaise, the diagnosis of xanthogranulomatous pyelonephritis should be considered (17). Xanthogranulomatous pyelonephritis is usually secondary to a chronically obstructing staghorn calculus and is typically accompanied by a poorly functioning kidney.

Renal papillary necrosis may be due to a variety of disorders, including infection, diabetes, sickle cell disease, and analgesic abuse. Rarely, patients may present with acute ureteral obstruction from a sloughed papilla (18).

In patients with recurrent urinary tract infections, the presence of a foreign body or stone, especially struvite stones, may be the nidus of recurrent infections (19). A calculus in either the upper or lower urinary tract may act as a nidus for persistent infection or for continued pyuria despite antibiotics.

In patients with vague, long-standing urinary symptoms in the setting of sterile urine and without other identifiable causes, tuberculosis of the urinary tract should be considered. Urinary tract infection occurs via hematogenous spread of the organisms to the renal parenchyma initially. Spread to the collecting system may ensue; the renal pelvis, ureter, and bladder are sequentially infected (20).

In all patients with a urinary tract infection who do not respond appropriately to antibiotic therapy, imaging of the upper tract is useful for identifying complications (21). Complicated renal infection may be detected with ultrasound or CT (21). However, CT, particularly CT urography, is more sensitive and better depicts the extent of disease (21).

Trauma Trauma to the urinary tract, whether blunt, penetrating, or iatrogenic, is always considered serious in nature because the loss of a functioning kidney and even death are possible sequelae. Following blunt trauma to the upper urinary tract, the most common complaint is flank pain, and hematuria is usually present. All stable patients with post-traumatic hematuria require imaging of the upper urinary tract to exclude upper tract injury (22). CT is the modality of choice because it can be used to identify all grades of trauma and is the most sensitive test for detecting renal contusion, laceration, and hematoma, as well as identifying severe injuries such as renal fracture, renal artery occlusion, and ureteropelvic junction avulsion (23). CT urography has not been described in the literature as being useful in the setting of trauma, and therefore examples are not provided in this textbook. However, CT urography is likely to be useful in the future. All patients with suspected trauma should be imaged during both nephrographic and excretory phases of contrast material administration. The nephrographic phase evaluates parenchymal abnormalities, such as hematoma, contusion, and laceration; the excretory phase evaluates collecting system injury. In patients with severe obstruction, the collecting system may not be opacified. In these cases, a distinct transition point of hydroureter may be present on CT. In patients with ureteral transection, a urinoma is typically present (24).

Congenital Abnormalities CT urography is useful for detecting abnormalities in the number and location of kidneys as well as variants in the intrarenal collecting system and ureteral anatomy. For example, horseshoe and pelvic kidneys may be detected using CT in almost all cases (25,26). CT urography provides multiplanar and three-dimensional images that are useful for identifying the precise type of congenital anomaly.

Surgical Planning CT urography can be used to detect and stage urinary tract malignancies. The anatomic relationship of the kidneys, ureters, and bladder to adjacent structures may also be displayed for surgical planning. CT urography may be used to describe the size and location of renal masses prior to nephron-sparing surgery (27,28). Also, since CT can be used to describe the size and location of renal calculi, open, endoscopic, or extracorporeal management strategies may be planned.

HEMATURIA: DEFINITION AND DIAGNOSIS

Hematuria, whether gross or microscopic, may be a sign of urinary tract pathology. Gross hematuria is alarming to both the patient and the primary care provider and often leads to referral to a urologist. Whether and how to evaluate patients with microscopic hematuria is controversial in part because there is no consensus regarding the definition of microscopic hematuria. Also, a small percentage of the normal population has microscopic hematuria. Thus, the American Urologic Association commissioned a panel to formulate best practice guidelines on asymptomatic microscopic hematuria. This document is used here to review our recommendations (29).

Definition Gross hematuria is defined as the detection of blood in the urine with the unaided eye from either a voided or a catheterized specimen. Microscopic hematuria is not as simply defined. Several factors contribute to the definition of microscopic hematuria, including the urine collection method, hematuria detection method, number of positive results, and patient characteristics.

Urinalysis for the detection of microscopic hematuria should be collected in one of two ways—by a fresh-voided, midstream, "clean-catch" urine sample or by sterile catheterization (29). The second may be reserved for patients who are obese, patients with phimosis or other anatomical reasons for potential contamination, or patients whose previous samples were contaminated as noted by the presence of squamous epithelial cells on microscopic analysis. Urine samples should not be contaminated with oxidizing agents such as betadine because this may lead to a false-positive dipstick analysis (30).

Detection of microscopic blood in the urine is most simply performed with a urinary dipstick. The urinary dipstick detects the presence of hemoglobin, either free or within red blood cells (RBCs), by an oxidation reaction with substances present on the dipstick resulting in a change in color (30). The sensitivity of dipstick urinalysis is between 91% and 100% (31), but its specificity in detecting less than five RBCs per high power field is between 65% and 99% (32,33). The chamber count and sediment count both confirm the presence of hematuria because the dipstick test may detect myoglobin. They can also be used to quantitate the number of RBCs. Although the chamber count may be more accurate, the American Urological Association Best Practice Policy Panel recommends using the sediment count (29). The sediment count involves centrifugation of 10 ml of urine for 5 minutes at 2,000 rpm (34). The pellet is resuspended in 0.5 to 1 ml of supernatant and analyzed

under a microscope. The presence of at least three RBCs per high power field is considered positive (29).

Although a urine sediment containing at least three RBCs per high power field is considered positive, characteristics of the patient determine if an additional urine sediment analysis should be performed or if the patient should be evaluated further. If a patient has any one of several risk factors associated with an increased likelihood of malignancy or other significant disease in the urinary tract (Table 1.1), it is recommended that a full evaluation of both the upper and lower urinary tract be performed on the basis of only one positive urinalysis (29). In low-risk patients (i.e., patients without risk factors), a complete workup is indicated only when three RBCs per high power field are found on two of three properly obtained samples (29). However, a single negative urinalysis does not preclude the absence of significant urinary tract disease.

Prevalence Multiple population-based screening studies have been performed to assess the prevalence of asymptomatic microscopic hematuria among adults. The five largest studies found the prevalence to be between 0.18% and 33% (33). The positive predictive value of microscopic hematuria in seven non-population-based studies in which patients had microscopic hematuria and a full workup was between 3.4% and 81.0%, with most studies noting a positive predictive value in the 20% to 30% range (33).

Evaluation The evaluation of a patient with microscopic hematuria includes a thorough history and physical examination. Low-risk patients with a history of vigorous exercise, trauma, menstruation, sexual activity, viral illness, or infection rarely need a complete workup. Laboratory testing should include a serum creatinine. The urine should be collected for 24 hours if 1+ or more proteinuria exists on the dipstick. Patients with significant proteinuria, dysmorphic RBC or red cell casts, or elevated serum creatinine should be

Table 1.1. Risk factors for significant disease in patients with microscopic hematuria[a]

Smoking history
Occupational exposure to chemicals or dyes (benzenes or aromatic amines)
History of gross hematuria
Age >40 years
Previous urologic history
History of irritative voiding symptoms
History of urinary tract infection
Analgesic abuse (e.g., phenacetin)
History of pelvic irradiation
Cyclophosphamide

[a]From Grossfeld GD, Litwin MS, Wolf, JS, et al. Evaluation of asymptomatic microscopic hematuria in adults: the American Urological Association best practice policy—part I: definition, detection, prevalence, and etiology. *Urology*. 2001;57:599–603.

considered for evaluation for glomerular or tubulointerstitial disease. Unexplained hematuria should be approached as follows: all patients with two of three urine sediments containing three or more RBCs per high power field or high-risk patients with a single positive urine sediment require evaluation of both the upper tract (kidneys, intrarenal collecting system, and ureters) and lower tract (bladder and urethra) to determine the cause of hematuria. A complete evaluation includes cytology, cystoscopy, and upper tract imaging.

Cytology Urinary cytology is an essential component in the workup of microscopic hematuria. Transitional cells are frequently sloughed into the urine and may be analyzed microscopically for the presence of cytologic abnormalities. A voided, clean-catch specimen should be obtained. Bladder barbotage, or washings, may have a higher yield; however, one study showed no statistically significant difference between the two (35). Urinary cytology had a sensitivity of 38% and a specificity of 98.3%, with a noted increase in sensitivity with increased malignancy grade (35). Use of ImmunoCyt, an assay that consists of a mixture of monoclonal antibodies that react to tumor markers of transitional cell carcinoma, has increased the sensitivity of tumor detection when combined with urinary cytology. In a multicenter prospective trial, overall sensitivity of urinary cytology was 17.9%, 46.3%, and 63.8%, respectively, for grade 1, grade 2, and grade 3 transitional cell carcinoma, whereas the sensitivity of ImmunoCyt was 60.7%, 75.6%, and 76.8%, respectively. The sensitivity of the combined tests was 66.7%, 78%, and 87%, respectively (36).

Cystoscopy Cystoscopic evaluation of the urethra and bladder is another important component in the evaluation of hematuria. Cystoscopy may be performed with a rigid cystoscope, with complete evaluation of the mucosal surface, trigone, ureteral orifices, bladder neck, and urethra. The advent of the flexible cystoscope has allowed urologists to perform an equally thorough examination in the office setting with less patient discomfort. Red flat patches of mucosa generally indicate carcinoma in situ; papillary lesions often represent transitional cell carcinoma.

Upper Tract Imaging Imaging of the upper tract is required for the complete workup of hematuria because lesions in the kidneys or ureters may be the source of blood in the urine. Several imaging modalities can be used to image the upper tracts; each has advantages and disadvantages. CT urography is the most comprehensive imaging evaluation of the urinary tract; however, its role in the evaluation of patients with hematuria and other disorders can be understood better after a brief review of other modalities. In general, CT urography provides an evaluation of all major anatomic portions of the urinary tract except the urethra and prostate gland. However, CT urography requires IV injection of iodinated contrast material and utilizes ionizing radiation.

Ultrasound Ultrasound is a safe, noninvasive, and informative evaluation of the kidneys, and it does not utilize ionizing radiation. Ultrasound is a good examination of the kidneys for masses. However, ultrasound is not as sensitive as CT in detecting renal masses. Ultrasound, compared to CT, is able to identify 26% of masses <1 cm, 60% of masses between 1 and 2 cm, 82% of masses between 2 and 3 cm, and 85% of masses >3 cm (37). The advantages of ultrasound are its ability to differentiate renal cysts from renal tumors and its ability to detect hydronephrosis, which usually indicates obstruction in adults. In addition, Doppler ultrasound allows for dynamic flow images of the renal vessels to diagnose various vascular disease states and obstruction.

Although renal ultrasound is able to detect upper tract obstruction, the cause of the obstruction must be inferred from secondary signs. For example, in patients with renal colic, ultrasound findings of hydronephrosis, hydroureter, stones, and the absence of urine flow from the ipsilateral ureter are diagnostic of ureteral obstruction with a sensitivity as high as 96.3% and specificity of 100% (38). A change in resistive index of 0.04 or greater in patients with unilateral renal colic has a specificity of 100% and sensitivity of 96% for acute unilateral obstruction (39). However, ultrasound detection of calculi is poor, yielding a sensitivity of 24% and a specificity of 90% (40). The inability to adequately visualize the full course of the ureter limits its ability to detect many causes of urinary tract obstruction.

It has been suggested that the upper tract should be evaluated with ultrasound alone in patients with microscopic hematuria (34); however, several studies indicate that ultrasound alone is insufficient. In a prospective analysis of patients with hematuria, both IVU and ultrasound were performed in the evaluation of the upper tracts. Ultrasound alone missed 42% of upper tract neoplasms, whereas IVU missed 27% of them, leading the authors to recommend combining ultrasound and IVU in the evaluation of patients with hematuria (40). The limitations of ultrasound in the evaluation of the urinary tract in patients with hematuria again stem from the fact that ultrasound cannot be used to evaluate the entirety of the ureters; abdominal bowel gas blocks the path of ultrasound such that a sonographic "window" cannot be obtained.

Intravenous Urography Prior to the introduction of CT urography, IVU had been considered the best initial imaging test for the evaluation of hematuria. In addition, relative to cross-sectional imaging modalities, IVU was inexpensive and widely available. IVU allowed for detection of both renal parenchymal masses and lesions of the urinary collecting system and bladder, including intraluminal and urothelial lesions. Additional advantages of IVU included the ability to assess differential renal function, estimate the degree of obstruction, localize calculi, and depict anatomy that allowed for surgical planning (41,42). However, IVU could not be used to distinguish cystic from solid renal masses and had a poor sensitivity in the detection of small (≤3cm) masses (39). Compared to CT, the sensitivity of IVU in the detection of renal masses <2 cm, between 2 and 3 cm, and >3 cm was found to be only 21%, 52%, and 85%, respectively (40). Regarding the ability of IVU to diagnose the cause of microscopic hematuria, in one study abnormalities were diagnosed with a sensitivity of 60.5% and specificity of 97.4% (43); the sensitivity for direct visualization of ureteral stones was 52% to 81% (44,45). Additional drawbacks of IVU have included difficulty visualizing radiolucent stones and differentiating them from tumors, the necessity of obtaining delayed films in the setting of severe obstruction, contrast material-induced nephrotoxicity and other reactions (41), and dependence on renal function for adequate opacification of the renal parenchyma and collecting system.

Retrograde Pyelography Retrograde pyelography has historically been regarded as the most sensitive examination of the intrarenal collecting system and ureters. In contrast to IVU, retrograde pyelography may be performed in patients with abnormal renal function because opacification of the upper tracts is not dependent on renal excretion. In addition, retrograde pyelography does not require IV injection of contrast material; therefore, contrast material reactions are rare. However, retrograde pyelography requires catheterization of the urethra, bladder, and distal ureters, and general anesthesia may be needed in most patients.

CT Urography CT urography has become the most useful imaging test of the urinary tract. It provides a single noninvasive examination of the kidneys, ureters, and bladder in one test. As a result, CT urography is the current modality of choice for evaluation of painless gross or microscopic hematuria. CT urography allows for identification of stones, renal parenchymal masses, and urothelial abnormalities.

In the detection of pathology among patients with microscopic hematuria, CT has also been established as superior to both ultrasound and IVU. In 86 patients with microscopic hematuria and a negative IVU, CT was used to diagnose conclusively the cause of hematuria; diagnoses included 39 inflammatory lesions, 26 calculi, nine malignant neoplasms, five vascular anomalies, four benign masses, and three infarcts (46). In a prospective comparison of CT to IVU in the evaluation of microscopic hematuria, CT had a sensitivity of 100% and specificity of 97.4%, with an overall accuracy of 98.3% in determining the cause for hematuria (43). Furthermore, CT was used to diagnose incidental, nonurinary abdominal or pelvic disease in 40 of 115 patients, all of which were not detected with IVU.

CT has long been the preferred modality for the detection and characterization of renal masses, but one of its greatest benefits (compared to IVU or ultrasound) is in the classification of small renal masses and renal cysts. In two series comparing CT features to pathologic findings in renal masses 3 cm or less, several CT findings correlated with malignant pathological features. In addition, among cystic lesions, CT correctly identified thick or nodular fibrous capsule with a specificity of 78% and sensitivity of 67% (47). CT and ultrasound detection rates of different sized lesions were respectively as follows: 0 to 5 mm, 47% and 0%; 5 to 10 mm, 60% and 21%; 10 to 15 mm, 75% and 28%; 15 to 20 mm, 100% and 58%; 20 to 25 mm, 100% and 79%; and

25 to 30 mm, 100% and 100% (48). In addition, CT is accurate in staging of renal cell carcinomas, correctly diagnosing stage I renal cell carcinomas with 96% sensitivity and 93% specificity (49). The Bosniak classification system of CT findings has allowed radiologists to accurately characterize cystic renal masses as benign or malignant (50).

Regarding urothelial neoplasms, although CT urography shows promise, test characteristics have not been fully studied. In one series, 15 of 16 urothelial malignancies were identified at CT urography—six in the renal pelvis and ureters and nine in the bladder (26). In a second series, 18 of 27 upper tract neoplasms were identified prospectively and 24 were detected retrospectively. Interestingly, three-dimensional reformations only detected 6 of 27 neoplasms (51). The role of CT urography in staging urothelial malignancies remains to be determined. The accuracy of CT in staging upper tract transitional cell carcinoma was 59.5% in one study; 16.2% of patients were understaged (52).

MRI Although not the primary examination for hematuria, MRI has been found useful in select patient populations in whom CT urography is relatively contraindicated. These include children, pregnant women, patients with an allergy to iodinated contrast media, and patients with renal insufficiency. Also, MRI may be helpful in staging renal cancers and in the evaluation of the indeterminate cystic renal mass. In one study, MRI was used to identify more septations or nodularity than CT (53). MRI was used to reclassify 7 of 69 cystic renal masses, resulting in more aggressive management (53). Using protocols that display the renal collecting systems and ureters, MRI can image the upper tract urothelium; however, small caliceal abnormalities are not well-delineated with MRI (54).

MRI does not detect calculi as well as CT (55). Therefore, MRI is typically used in patients in whom CT is relatively contraindicated. MRI can be considered in patients with indinavir stones. Indinavir is a drug used to treat patients with HIV infection. The stones that may develop can be visualized with MRI and not with unenhanced CT in some patients (56). Overall, MR urography shows promise but lags behind CT urography. Furthermore, MRI is more expensive and less readily available.

SUMMARY

Although all imaging modalities play an important role in imaging the urinary tract, CT urography represents the most comprehensive imaging examination of the urinary tract. It has replaced conventional IV urography in some academic centers. To guide physicians on the relative merits of the imaging modalities, the American College of Radiology developed criteria for determining appropriate imaging examinations for diagnosis and treatment for the evaluation of hematuria (Appendix 1) and acute flank pain (Appendix 2). As imaging technology continues to mature, it is expected that CT urography will play an increasingly important role in the evaluation of the urinary tract.

APPENDIX 1[a]

MAJOR RECOMMENDATIONS

ACR Appropriateness Criteria[a]

Clinical condition: Hematuria

Variant 1: All patients except those with generalized renal parenchymal disease or young females with hemorrhagic cystitis.

Radiologic Exam Procedure	Appropriateness Rating	Comments
X-ray, kidney, intravenous urography, IVP	8	
CT, kidney, urography	8	
US, kidney and bladder, transabdominal	6	May miss ureteral and urothelial lesions; abdomen x-ray, retrograde pyelography, and cystoscopy are useful adjuncts.
X-ray, kidney, pyelography retrograde	5	
MRI, kidney, urography	4	
CT, abdomen and pelvis	4	CT may follow IVP or US if initial findings are ambiguous.
Intervention, kidney, angiography	4	Rarely, vascular malformations may cause hematuria and require angiography for diagnosis.
X-ray, abdomen, KUB	2	It is assumed that an abdomen film will be part of the indicated IVP. If an IVP is not performed, KUB may be performed along with US.
MRI, abdomen and pelvis	2	
Urinary tract scintigraphy	2	
Virtual cystoscopy	2	
Appropriateness Criteria Scale **1 2 3 4 5 6 7 8 9** **1 = Least appropriate; 9 = Most appropriate**		

Variant 2: Due to generalized renal parenchymal disease.

Radiologic Exam Procedure	Appropriateness Rating	Comments
US, kidney and bladder, transabdominal	8	For renal volume and morphology and as localizer for biopsy.
X-ray, chest	6	For cardiopulmonary and pleural manifestations of renal diseases.
X-ray, kidney, pyelography retrograde	3	
CT abdomen and pelvis	2	Routine
Intervention, kidney, angiography	2	
MRI, abdomen and pelvis	2	
Urinary tract scintigraphy	2	
CT, kidney, urography	2	
MRI, kidney, urography	2	
CT, bladder, high resolution, virtual cystoscopy	2	
X-ray, abdomen, KUB	1	
X-ray, kidney, intravenous urography, IVP	1	
Appropriateness Criteria Scale **1 2 3 4 5 6 7 8 9** **1 = Least appropriate; 9 = Most appropriate**		

Variant 3: Hemorrhagic cystitis in females less than 40 years old (hematuria completely clears with therapy).

Radiologic Exam Procedure	Appropriateness Rating	Comments
CT abdomen and pelvis	2	This and other imaging are rarely needed for diagnosis. Routine.
Urinary tract scintigraphy	2	
MRI, abdomen, pelvis	2	
Intervention, kidney, angiography	2	
CT, kidney, urography	2	
MRI, kidney, urography	2	
X-ray, pyelography retrograde	2	
CT, kidney, high resolution, virtual cystoscopy	2	
X-ray, kidney, intravenous urography, IVP	1	
X-ray, abdomen, KUB	1	
US, kidney and bladder, transabdominal	1	
Appropriateness Criteria Scale **1 2 3 4 5 6 7 8 9** **1 = Least appropriate; 9 = Most appropriate**		

[a]From Choyke PL, Bluth EI, Bush WH Jr, et al. *Expert Panel on Urologic Imaging. Radiologic investigation of patients with hematuria.* Available at www.acr.org/s_acr/bin.asp?CID=1202&DID=11827&DOC=FILE.PDF. Reston, VA: American College of Radiology, 2005. Reprinted with permission of the American College of Radiology. No other representation of this material is authorized without express, written permission from the American College of Radiology.

APPENDIX 2[a]

MAJOR RECOMMENDATIONS

ACR Appropriateness Criteria[a]
Clinical condition: Acute onset flank pain
Variant 1: Suspicion of stone disease.

Radiologic Exam Procedure	Appropriateness Rating	Comments
X-ray, kidney, intravenous urography, IVP	8	
CT, kidney, helical, without contrast	8	
US, renal, with Doppler and KUB	6	Preferred exam in pregnant and allergic patients.
MRI, kidney	4	
X-ray, abdomen, KUB	1	Most useful in patients with known stone disease.
Appropriateness Criteria Scale **1 2 3 4 5 6 7 8 9** **1 = Least appropriate; 9 = Most appropriate**		

[a]From Choyke PL, Bluth EI, Bush WH Jr, et al. *Expert Panel on Urologic Imaging. Radiologic investigation of patients with hematuria.* Available at www.acr.org/s_acr/bin.asp?CID=1202&DID=11827&DOC=FILE.PDF. Reston, VA: American College of Radiology, 2005. Reprinted with permission of the American College of Radiology. No other representation of this material is authorized without express, written permission from the American College of Radiology.

REFERENCES

1. Swain J. The effect of the roentgen rays on calculi; with the report of renal calculus in which the diagnosis was confirmed by skiagraphy. *Bristol Med Chirurgical J.* 1897;15:1–13.

2. Swick M. Intravenous urography by means of the sodium salt of 5 iodo-2-pyridon-n-acetic acid. *JAMA.* 1930;95:1403.

3. Goldman SM, Sandler CM. Genitourinary imaging: the past 40 years. *Radiology.* 2000;215:313–324.

4. Bosniak MA. Nephrotomography: a relatively unappreciated but extremely valuable diagnostic tool. *Radiology.* 1974;113:313–324.

5. Fielding JR, Steele G, Fox LA, et al. Spiral computerized tomography in the evaluation of acute flank pain: a replacement for excretory urography. *J Urol.* 1997;157:2071–2073.

6. Jayson M, Sanders H. Increased incidence of serendipitously discovered renal cell carcinoma. *Urology.* 1998;51:203–205.

7. Hanna JK. Antenatal hydronephrosis and ureteropelvic junction obstruction: the case for early intervention. *Urology.* 2000;55:612–615.

8. Nixon HH. Hydronephrosis in children: a clinical study of seventy-eight cases with special reference to the role of aberrant renal vessels and the results of conservative operations. *Br J Surg.* 1953;40:601–604.

9. Bateson E, Atkinson D. Circumcaval ureter: a new classification. *Clin Radiol.* 1969;20:173–177.

10. Schlussel RN, Retik AB. Ectopic ureter, ureterocele, and other anomalies of the ureter. In: Walsh PC, Retik AB, Vaughn ED, et al., eds. *Campbell's urology.* 8th ed. Philadelphia: Saunders; 2002: 2007–2052.

11. Gulmi FA, Felsen D, Vaughn ED. Pathophysiology of urinary tract obstruction. In: Walsh PC, Retik AB, Vaughn ED, et al., eds. *Campbell's urology.* 8th ed. Philadelphia: Saunders; 2002:411–462.

12. Sosa R, Vaughan EJ, Gibbons R. *Retroperitoneal fibrosis.* AUA update series VI, lesson 21. 1987.

13. Linblad B, Almgren B, Bergqvist D, et al. Abdominal aortic aneurysm with perianeurysmal fibrosis: experience from 11 Swedish vascular centers. *J Vasc Surg.* 1991;13:231–237.

14. Hulnick DH, Megibow AJ, Balthazar EJ, et al. Computed tomography in the evaluation of diverticulitis. *Radiology.* 1948;152:491–495.

15. Huang JJ, Tseng CC. Emphysematous pyelonephritis: clinicoradiological classification, management, prognosis, and pathogenesis. *Arch Intern Med.* 2000;160:797–805.

16. St Lezin M, Hoffmann R, Stroller ML. Pyonephrosis: diagnosis and treatment. *Br J Urol.* 1992;70:360–363.

17. Malek RS, Elder JS. Xanthogranulomatous pyelonephritis: a critical analysis of 26 cases and of the literature. *J Urol.* 1978;119:589–593.

18. Bach PH, Thanh NTK. Penal papillary necrosis—40 years on. *Toxicol Pathol.* 1998;40:73–91.

19. Neu HC. Urinary tract infections. *Am J Med.* 1991;92:63S–70S.

20. Johnson WD Jr, Johnson CW, Lowe FC. Tuberculosis and parasitic disease of the genitourinary system. In: Walsh PC, Retik AB, Vaughn ED, et al., eds. *Campbell's urology.* 8th ed. Philadelphia: Saunders; 2002:743–763.

21. Kaplan DM, Rosenfield AT, Smith RC. Advances in the imaging of renal infection. Helical CT and modern coordinated imaging. *Infect Dis Clin North Am.* 1997;11:681–705.

22. Miller KS, McAninch JW. Radiographic assessment of renal trauma: our 15-year experience. *J Urol.* 1995;154:352–355.

23. Kenney PJ, Panicek DM, Witanowski LS. Computed tomography of ureteral disruption. *J Comput Assist Tomogr.* 1987;3:480–484.

24. Titton RL, Gervais DA, Hahn PF, et al. Urine leaks and urinomas: diagnosis and imaging-guided intervention. *Radiographics.* 2003;23: 1133–1147.

25. Aljabri B, MacDonald PS, Satin R, et al. Incidence of major venous and renal anomalies relevant to aortoiliac surgery as demonstrated by computed tomography. *Ann Vasc Surg.* 2001;15:615–618.

26. Caoili EM, Cohan RH, Korobkin M, et al. Urinary tract abnormalities: initial experience with multi-detector row CT urography. *Radiology.* 2002;222:353–360.

27. Uzzo RG, Novick AC. Nephron sparing surgery for renal tumors: indications, techniques and outcomes. *J Urol.* 2001;166:6–18.

28. Halpern EJ, Mitchell DG, Wechsler RJ, et al. Preoperative evaluation of living renal donors: comparison of CT angiography and MR angiography. *Radiology.* 2000;216:434–439.

29. Grossfeld GD, Litwin MS, Wolf JS, et al. Evaluation of asymptomatic microscopic hematuria in adults: the American Urological Association best practice policy—Part I: definition, detection, prevalence, and etiology. *Urology.* 2001;57:599–603.

30. Corwin HL, Silverstein MD. Microscopic hematuria. *Clin Lab Med.* 1988;8:601–610.

31. Sutton JM. Evaluation of hematuria in adults. *JAMA.* 1989;262: 1214–1219.

32. Mariani AJ, Luangphinith S, Loo S, et al. Dipstick chemical urinalysis: an accurate cost-effective screening test. *J Urol.* 1984;132:64–66.

33. Woolhandler S, Pels RJ, Bor DH, et al. Dipstick urinalysis screening of asymptomatic adults for urinary tract disorders. I. Hematuria and proteinuria. *JAMA.* 1989;262:1214–1219.

34. Corwin HL, Silverstein MD. The diagnosis of neoplasia in patients with asymptomatic microscopic hematuria: a decision analysis. *J Urol.* 1988;139:1002–1006.

35. Planz B, Jochims E, Deix T, et al. The role of urinary cytology for detection of bladder cancer. *Eur J Surg Oncol.* 2005;31:304–308.

36. Pfister C, Chautard D, Devonec M, et al. Immunocyte test improves the diagnostic accuracy of urinary cytology: results of a French multicenter study. *J Urol.* 2003;169:921–924.

37. Warshauer DM, McCarthy SM, Street L, et al. Detection of renal masses: sensitivities and specificities of exrectory urogram/linear tomography, US and CT. *Radiology.* 1988;169:363–365.

38. Soyer P, Levesque M, Lecloirec A, et al. Evaluation of the role of echography in the positive diagnosis of renal colic secondary to kidney stone. *J Radiol.* 1990;71:445–450.

39. Shokeir AA, Abdulmaabound M. Prospective comparison of nonenhanced helical computerized tomography and Doppler ultrasonography for the diagnosis of renal colic. *J Urol.* 2001;165:1085–1084.

40. Fowler KA, Locken JA, Duchesne JH, et al. US for detecting renal calculi with nonenhanced CT as a reference standard. *Radiology.* 2002;222:109–113.

41. Khadra MH, Pickard RS, Charlton M, et al. A prospective analysis of 1,930 patients with hematuria to evaluate current diagnostic practice. *J Urol.* 2000;163:524–527.

42. Heidenreich A, Desgrandschamps F, Terrier F, et al. Modern approach of diagnosis and management of acute flank pain: review of all imaging modalities. *Eur Urol.* 2002;41:351–362.

43. Gray Sears CL, Ward JF, Sears ST, et al. Prospective comparison of computerized tomography and excretory urography in the initial evaluation of asymptomatic microhematuria. *J Urol.* 2002;168:2457–2460.

44. Roth CS, Bowyer BA, Bergquist TH. Utility of the plain abdominal radiograph for diagnosing ureteral calculi. *Ann Emerg Med.* 1985;14:311–315.

45. Ruppert-Kohlmayr AJ, Stacher R, Preidler KW, et al. Native spiral computerized tomography in patients with acute flank pain—yes or no? *Fortschr Roentgenstr.* 1999;170:168–173.

46. Lang EK, Macchia RJ, Thomas R, et al. Improved detection of renal pathologic features on multiphase helical CT compared with IVU in patients presenting with microscopic hematuria. *Urology.* 2003;61: 528–532.

47. Silverman SG, Lee BY, Seltzer SE, et al. Small (≤3 cm) renal masses: correlation of spiral CT features and pathologic findings. *Am J Roentgenol.* 1994;163:597–605.

48. Jamis-Dow CA, Choyke PL, Jennings SB, et al. Small (< or = 3-cm) renal masses: detection with CT versus US and pathologic correlation. *Radiology.* 1996;198:785–788.

49. Catalano C, Fraiolo F, Laghi A, et al. High-resolution multidetector CT in the preoperative evaluation of patients with renal cell carcinoma. *Am J Roentgenol.* 2003;180:1271–1277.

50. Bosniak MA. Diagnosis and management of patients with complicated cystic lesions of the kidney. *Am J Roentgenol.* 1997;169:819–821.

51. Caoili E, Cohan RH, Inampudi P, et al. MDCT urography of upper tract neoplasms. *Am J Roentgenol.* 2005;184:1873–1881.

52. Scolieri MJ, Paik ML, Brown SL, et al. Limitations of computed tomography in the preoperative staging of upper tract urothelial carcinoma. *Urology.* 2000;56:930–934.

53. Israel GM, Hindman N, Bosniak MA. Evaluation of cystic renal masses; comparison of CT and MR imaging by using the Bosniak classification system. *Radiology.* 2004;231:365–371.

54. Nolte-Ernsting CCA, Bucker A, Adam GB, et al. Gadolinium-enhanced excretory MR urography after low-dose diuretic injection: comparison with conventional excretory urography. *Radiology.* 1998;209: 147–157.

55. Sudah M, Vanninen R, Partanen K, et al. Patients with acute flank pain: comparison of MR urography with unenhanced helical CT. *Radiology.* 2002;223:98–105.

56. Hermans BP, Materne R, Marot JC, et al. Indinavir calculi: diagnosis with magnetic resonance urography. *Eur Urol.* 2000;37:634–635.

CHAPTER TWO
CT UROGRAPHY TECHNIQUES

RICHARD H. COHAN, MD

ELAINE M. CAOILI, MD

The optimal technique for performing CT urography (CTU) has not been defined. However, more information is emerging that should contribute to improvements in the way in which this study is performed. In this chapter, a variety of issues related to the proper performance of CTU are discussed. There is a brief review of the recent developments of CTU, with an emphasis on the emergence and importance of the axial excretory phase CT acquisition. Variations in protocols, including differences in the timing of excretory phase acquisition and use of three-phase and split bolus approaches, are reviewed. Urinary tract segment nonopacification is discussed as well as ways to minimize this problem. The potential benefits of ancillary techniques, such as turning or exercising the patient between the initiation of the contrast material injection and excretory phase image acquisition, abdominal compression, saline hydration, and administration of diuretics, in improving urinary tract distention and opacification and, hopefully, lesion detection are also addressed. It is hoped that after reading this chapter the reader will have gained enough knowledge to contribute actively to the further refinement of this technique.

EVOLUTION OF CTU

Combining CT and Intravenous Urography (Hybrid Studies) One of the earliest descriptions of using CT to assist in evaluation of the urinary tract involved combining CT and intravenous urography (IVU) (1). Using this approach, patients were evaluated initially with plain radiography and linear tomography. Contrast material was then injected intravenously, during which time a standard intravenous urogram was obtained. Subsequently, the patient was transferred to a CT suite, at which time delayed enhanced CT images were obtained through the kidneys. With this approach, the purpose of the CT images was to identify small renal lesions that would have been missed if only an intravenous urogram was performed.

Although this technique likely improved study sensitivity in detecting renal masses over that of IVU, there were two limitations. First, it is not always easy to transfer a patient quickly from a conventional x-ray room onto a CT scanner. Essentially, both rooms must be vacant at some point for the transfer to occur, which is not always easily done in a busy radiology department. Second, renal masses are not evaluated fully; the delayed enhanced CT images are not obtained during the nephrographic phase of renal enhancement—the phase that is most ideal for detecting renal masses. More important, an unenhanced CT is not obtained. Therefore, renal masses cannot be evaluated for enhancement.

Hybrid CT/IVU: CT Room Modification As an alternative, a CT suite may be modified by adding conventional x-ray equipment to a CT scanner (2). This modification allows patients to have conventional radiographs obtained while they remain on the CT table. Preliminary results

with this approach were encouraging because now CT evaluation of the renal parenchyma could be obtained at any time (3). This approach is also predicated on the belief that the excretory phase is imaged better with radiography than with CT. Axial CT images are not obtained routinely after excretion of contrast material into the renal collecting systems and ureters has occurred, even though studies have suggested that excretory phase conventional radiography is probably not as accurate as are excretory phase axial images. Also, adopting this hybrid technique requires substantial additional expenditure.

Nevertheless, there have been a number of investigations in which the CT digital (or scan projection) radiograph was used to assess the urinary tract instead of conventional radiographs. Enhanced digital CT radiographs were then developed that appeared similar to conventional radiographs and were as sensitive as radiographs in detecting urinary tract abnormalities, including urolithiasis (4). Thus, the CT scanner could be used to obtain intravenous urography-like images without the need for CT room alterations. As with all projection-type techniques, however, with digital radiography the urinary tract can be obscured by overlying structures, such as gas-filled loops of bowel. As a result, bowel preparation may be helpful when this method of excretory phase urinary tract imaging is employed.

Using Axial Images to Evaluate the Renal Collecting Systems, Ureters, and Bladder Concurrently, several investigators began to utilize thin section axial images rather than conventional radiographs to evaluate the urinary tract in its entirety (5–7). In comparison to conventional or digital radiography, axial images would not be affected by overlying structures, making bowel preparation unnecessary. However, this approach required a paradigm shift. It had been thought that urothelial abnormalities could not be detected on axial CT images due to their decreased resolution compared with IVU (3). However, with the introduction of multidetector row CT, it became possible to obtain thin section images of the entire urinary tract during a single breath-hold, permitting one to create high spatial resolution images of the urothelium in multiple planes. Preliminary results suggested that, in fact, CTU performed with this approach, generally termed multidetector or multislice CTU, was effective in detecting both benign and malignant urinary tract pathology (6). Small abnormalities, such as renal tubular ectasia, papillary necrosis, and even tiny (2- or 3-mm maximal diameter) urothelial cancers, could be identified. Thus, it was suggested that multidetector CTU could replace IVU and the combined IVU–CT hybrid studies (6,8).

It has become apparent that CTU obtained with thin section excretory phase axial images (generally acquired using a thickness of 2.5 mm or less) is more sensitive in detecting urinary tract pathology than digital scout images or conventional excretory urographic images. The advantages of the axial CT approach are best seen in its ability to detect urothelial cancers and ureteritis. IVU and digital scout CT images only image the lumina of the renal collecting systems, ureters, and bladder. They cannot be used to visualize their walls. Although it has been assumed that abnormalities of the urinary tract that affect the urothelium nearly always affect the lumen, this is now known not to be the case. Occasional urothelial malignancies and some cases of ureteritis and cystitis can produce pronounced urothelial wall thickening and yet have little or no effect on the diameter or the morphology of the renal collecting system, ureteral, or bladder lumen. Circumferential wall thickening can be identified on axial CT images when it is undetectable on digital CT images, IVU, and even retrograde pyelography (6,8). For this reason, some early advocates of the combined IVU–CT approach have recently converted to a CTU technique that relies only on axial images to assess the urothelium.

TECHNIQUES OF AXIAL IMAGE CTU

Single Bolus Technique Two different approaches in performing axial image CTU have evolved. The most comprehensive imaging protocol utilizes at least three different image acquisitions: unenhanced scans to assess the kidneys and ureters for calculi and to assist in characterization of any subsequently detected renal masses; early enhanced nephrographic phase scans for optimal detection and characterization of renal masses (commenced after injection of a single bolus of contrast material has been administered); and delayed excretory phase images for evaluation of the renal collecting systems, ureters, and bladder (7,9). Although some have added more series, such as arterial, corticomedullary phase (10,11), and additional excretory phase images (6), these are not obtained routinely.

A variety of different image thicknesses have been utilized. In general, unenhanced images are obtained from the kidneys to the pubic symphysis using a reconstructed image thickness of 2.5 to 5 mm and no overlap. The nephrographic phase images are obtained utilizing the same reconstruction image thickness and interval but are performed either through the kidneys alone or through the entire abdomen. The latter approach allows for assessment of abnormalities outside the urinary tract, although enhancement of the liver is not optimal, since images are obtained after the portal venous phase. Despite this limitation, hepatic (and other nonrenal abdominal organs) enhancement is preferred during the nephrographic phase compared to the excretory phase due to improved sensitivity in detecting visceral organ abnormalities. It is important that multidetector CTU protocols include very thin section excretory phase images. Although an image thickness of 5 mm has occasionally been utilized (10), it is preferable for it to be no greater than 2.5 to 3.0 mm. Many researchers are reconstructing the original data set utilizing an image thickness of 0.625 to 1.25 mm (7,9). Reconstructions are then performed with no overlap if 0.625-mm-thick images are acquired. A 50% overlap can be used if thicker sections are obtained (5,9).

Contrast material injection involves administration of 100 to 150 ml of a 300 mg I/ml concentration of nonionic contrast material, which is administered by a mechanical injector at rates varying between 2 and 4 ml/sec (6,7). Since arterial phase images are not obtained routinely, more rapid injection rates are not required.

The recommended timing for each of the two contrast-enhanced phases has varied widely; however, nephrographic phase images are fairly consistently obtained 100 to 120 seconds after the administration of contrast material begins, provided that the contrast material is injected at the rates described in the previous text (6,7). There is less of a consensus about the timing of the excretory phase images. Excretory phase scans have been acquired between 3 (12) and 15 minutes (13) after the initiation of the contrast material injection. One reported series demonstrated that urinary tract abnormalities were more frequently detected when excretory phase images were obtained at 450 seconds compared with 300 seconds (14). Still another study found that urinary tract distention improved for up to 15 minutes after contrast injection began but then decreased (15). Based on these data, the optimal timing for excretory phase image acquisition appears to be between 7.5 and 15 minutes.

The three- or four-phase single bolus technique for CTU has been the most widely used (16). There is one important criticism, however: patients are exposed to more radiation in comparison with standard IVU. This criticism could be leveled at many CT protocols since CT scans inherently result in more radiation to the patient than does plain radiography.

Split Bolus Technique In 2001, two groups (5,17) reported on a different approach to performing CTU, in which administered contrast material was divided into two boluses. A sufficient delay was inserted between the two doses so that the patient would be imaged when the first dose was being excreted into the renal collecting systems, ureters, and bladder, while the second dose was still opacifying the renal parenchyma (5,17). With this approach, a single contrast-enhanced CT acquisition included both nephrographic and excretory phase images of the urinary tract, effectively eliminating the need for one of the contrast-enhanced CT acquisitions. The result was decreased patient radiation exposure compared with the three- or four-phase CTU protocols.

The split bolus protocol used by Chow and Sommer (5) is summarized as follows: first, 5-mm unenhanced images were obtained through the abdomen and pelvis, and then 40 ml of contrast material (300 mg I/ml) were injected at a rate of 2 ml/sec. After a delay of 2 minutes (during which time no scanning was performed), an additional 80 ml of contrast material (of the same concentration) were injected at the same rate. After a delay of an additional 1.5 minutes, CT scans were obtained of the abdomen and pelvis and reconstructed at 2.5-mm sections and 1.25-mm intervals. However, a net delay of 3.5 minutes between the first contrast material injection and the beginning of excretory phase image acquisition likely did not allow for maximal opacification and distention of the entire urinary tract. Therefore, a compression device was required. Images were obtained of the upper tract before and the lower tract after the compression device was released.

An alternative split bolus protocol was reported by another group (17). First, unenhanced CT scans were obtained of the abdomen and pelvis and reconstructed using 5-mm-thick sections and 5-mm intervals. Second, 30 ml of contrast material (300 mg I/ml) was administered by infusion rather than a power injector. After 15 minutes, the patient received an additional 100 ml of contrast material administered by a power injector at a rate of 2 ml/sec. After another 100 seconds, thin section images were acquired through the abdomen and pelvis (with images reconstructed contiguously using 5-mm thickness for axial image review but using a thickness of 2.5 mm and reconstruction interval of 1 mm for coronal reformatting). The total delay of more than 16.5 minutes was probably longer than desired for optimal urinary tract distention. Also, it is generally recommended that axial images be reviewed using a section thickness of <5 mm.

Kekelidze et al. (18) reported on their use of a triple bolus protocol whereby contrast material is administered at three different times and the patient is then imaged when the first bolus (30 ml of iodixanol 320) has been excreted, the second (50 ml of iodixanol 320), administered 7 minutes later, is in the renal parenchyma, and the third (65 ml of iodixanol 320), administered 2 minutes after that, opacifies the renal arteries. Using this protocol, the authors found that satisfactory images could be obtained.

The ability of the split bolus approach to eliminate one of the contrast-enhanced CT acquisitions has led to its adoption at many institutions. However, there are several theoretical limitations of the split bolus approach. First, the reduced volume of the first bolus may produce less distention and opacification of both the intrarenal collecting systems and the lower urinary tract, which could limit the ability to detect abnormalities. We have occasionally observed this to be a problem (19). Second, it has been reported that dense excreted contrast material in the renal collecting systems can create beam hardening-induced streak artifact that could limit evaluation of the renal parenchyma (20). Although it is unlikely that such artifact would prevent detection of a renal mass, it might preclude obtaining accurate attenuation measurements of renal masses that are adjacent to the collecting system, limiting characterization.

Finally, it must also be stressed that although the split bolus approach does reduce the radiation to which patients are exposed, the reduction is less than one-third that of the entire study. The highest dose component is the final thin section excretory phase. This phase is typically obtained with the thinnest collimation settings to maximize spatial resolution and, thereby, the detection of urothelial abnormalities. To counteract the increased noise caused by this thin collimation, the scanner dose is increased. The eliminated separate nephrographic phase series contributes

much less radiation because collimated settings are not as thin. Also, nephrographic phase images are usually only obtained through the kidneys or upper abdomen, whereas the other two series include the entire abdomen and pelvis. It could also be argued whether the modest decrease in radiation afforded by the split bolus technique is important when examining the elderly using CTU.

RADIATION REDUCTION BY LOWERING TUBE CURRENT

Patient radiation exposure during CTU can also be reduced by decreasing the dose technique used during individual series. Tube current or mA can be decreased substantially for unenhanced CT without compromising its ability to detect calculi (21,22), although the ideal amount by which the mA should be reduced has not been determined. Also, low mA settings may affect the accuracy of attenuation measurements of renal masses.

Degenhart and colleagues (23) evaluated the ability of low-mA CT to delineate opacified urinary tract segments during excretory phase imaging for CTU. The authors observed that "delineation" of the intrarenal collecting systems and proximal and mid ureters was comparable for standard-dose (176 mAs and 120 kVp) and low-dose (29 mAs and 120 kVp) techniques; however, the lower ureter was not seen as well with the low-dose technique. The authors concluded that CTU performed at the lower doses would have been unlikely to detect mucosal (and probably mural) lesions in the lower ureter. However, these results suggest that it might be possible to decrease the mA to a lesser extent without lowering sensitivity. Given that evaluation of the excretory phase images primarily involves comparing the very high attenuation opacified urine in the renal collecting systems and ureters to mucosal and mural abnormalities that are of considerably lower attenuation, successful mA reduction should theoretically be possible. An experimental study in pigs has, in fact, found that mAs can be decreased to 70 (but not below) without significantly decreasing image quality (24).

REDUCING RADIATION EXPOSURE BY ELIMINATING UNENHANCED SCANS

A radiation saving alternative to the split bolus approach is to eliminate the unenhanced phase. It could be argued that this phase may be unnecessary since renal and ureteral calculi might be identified on the nephrographic phase images and renal masses could be characterized by assessing them for de-enhancement (between the nephrographic and excretory phase images) rather than for enhancement (between unenhanced and nephrographic phase images).

Preliminary work has suggested, however, that one cannot rely exclusively on nephrographic and excretory phase scans to detect urinary tract calculi and to characterize renal masses. In one study, only 60% of urinary tract calculi seen on unenhanced images could be retrospectively detected on nephrographic or excretory phase images (25). These potentially missed calculi were small and obscured by contrast material that had already been excreted by the time the nephrographic phase scans were obtained. Furthermore, two of six solid malignant renal masses in this series did not de-enhance by more than 10 Hounsfield units in the 10.5-minutes between the nephrographic and excretory phase image acquisitions. These two masses did enhance by more than 10 Hounsfield units when unenhanced attenuation measurements were compared to measurements obtained on the nephrographic phase images.

Finally, if the low-mA technique is used during the unenhanced phase, the savings in radiation by not performing this initial series of images is small. For all of the previously mentioned reasons, elimination of the unenhanced scans is generally not recommended. However, this approach could still be considered in a select group of patients who are unlikely to have renal masses, whose recent previous imaging demonstrated no solid renal masses, or in whom detection of small calculi is not important.

UNOPACIFIED URINARY TRACT SEGMENTS

The most common problem encountered during CTU is lack of opacification of one or more urinary tract segments. This problem is usually seen in patients with nonobstructed systems (as a result of ureteral peristalsis), but it is also occasionally observed in patients with urinary tract obstruction.

Lack of urinary tract segment opacification has been noted on IVU examinations for years. When obstruction is the cause of nonvisualization on IVU, delayed films are usually obtained. In most patients, the obstructed system will gradually opacify over time, although this may take several hours. There is disagreement concerning the best way to deal with unopacified nonobstructed segments during IVU. Some advocate obtaining delayed films (particularly with the patient in the prone position), whereas others recommend performing fluoroscopy or even retrograde pyelography. Still others do not perform any additional imaging, believing that the vast majority of ureteral abnormalities, when present, will produce some type of abnormality besides nonopacification (usually dilatation) that will be visible during IVU.

Given the different approaches to segmental urinary tract nonopacification with IVU, it is not surprising that a variety of approaches are used during CTU. Approaches to the unopacified obstructed collecting system and unopacified nonobstructed segments are discussed separately.

The Unopacified or Partially Opacified Obstructed Urinary Tract The etiology of a complete or high-grade urinary tract obstruction is usually readily identified during CTU because excretion into the dilated renal collecting

system and ureter is not required for its visualization. Soft tissue attenuation urothelial neoplasms and blood clots, strictures, and calculi (which are almost always of high attenuation) may be visualized, particularly when outlined against water attenuation urine. For this reason, delayed imaging of the obstructed urinary tract is not required with CTU, which is another feature that makes CTU preferable to IVU.

A more interesting problem relates to the dependent layering of excreted contrast material in a dilated renal collecting system and ureter and in the normal-sized bladder in patients undergoing CTU. Contrast media has a higher specific gravity than urine. Thus, opacified urine tends to layer posteriorly in dilated systems or in the bladder. Abnormalities of the intrarenal collecting system and bladder walls adjacent to unopacified urine may still be detected (due to attenuation differences); however, in general, abnormalities are easier to detect when outlined by opacified urine. Thus, it is possible that layering compromises sensitivity in detecting at least some urinary tract pathology.

Some investigators (Nigel Cowan, personal communication) recommend having the patient ambulate between the initial contrast material injection and excretory phase acquisition. This may be done by first having the patient walk around the CT room and then by rotating the patient 360 degrees when he or she is placed back on the CT scanner table. Patient rotation alone is not always sufficient for optimal mixing of opacified and unopacified urine. After the patient is moved, he or she must be carefully repositioned on the CT scanner table (to ensure that subsequent imaging will include the entire urinary tract). Overall, these maneuvers require additional time and effort. We do not move the patient after contrast material injection for this reason. There is not sufficient proof or experience to show that the ability of CTU to detect urinary tract abnormalities is compromised significantly when the patient remains stationary throughout the study.

Another approach is to have the patient void immediately prior to the CTU exam. This minimizes the amount of unopacified urine in the bladder. The major drawback of this approach is that the bladder may not be distended at the time of excretory phase image acquisition unless a diuretic is employed.

The Incompletely Opacified Nonobstructed Urinary Tract A much more common problem concerns nonopacification of occasional nonobstructed urinary tract segments. Caoili et al. (26) observed that this problem was encountered frequently in the ureters but not in the intrarenal collecting system. Additionally, unopacified ureteral segments were more common distally than proximally. Although only 5% and 8% of proximal ureters had nonopacified segments in their series when imaged at 300 and 450 seconds, respectively, the percentages of unopacified segments increased dramatically for the distal ureters to 33% at 300 seconds and 24% at 450 seconds. These data suggest that nonopacification may be more of a problem when excretory phase images are obtained using shorter delays.

There are a number of possible responses to nonopacification. Some have added a second excretory phase series (in the hope that the same segment of ureter would not be unopacified on both series) (6). Others have supplemented the axial images with delayed CT scan projection radiographs so that ureteral segments not opacified on the axial images might be opacified at the time that the CT scan projection radiographs are obtained (27,28). One study demonstrated that addition of enhanced digital CT radiography increased the number of urinary tract segments that were completely opacified (28). In this series, the number of incompletely opacified urinary tract segments was reduced by more than 50% when axial image acquisition was followed by obtaining an enhanced CT scan projection radiograph 1 minute later, and as many as three additional CT scan projection radiographs at 2-minute intervals in cases in which all earlier images failed to demonstrate opacification of all segments.

Although this approach certainly has some advantages, it must be remembered that, like conventional radiography, CT scan projection radiographs only image the urinary tract lumen. Some mural abnormalities and probably occasional tiny filling defects projecting into the urinary tract lumen will be missed in segments that are opacified only on these images. Also, additional CT scan projection radiographs (or additional axial images) may not be uniformly successful. Some urinary tract segments will remain unopacified. Fortunately, the likelihood of a nonopacified normal-sized ureteral segment containing an abnormality is exceedingly low. Thus, although attempts should be made to minimize the number of unopacified ureteral segments, these segments can be assumed to be normal, with the understanding that there will be very rare false-negative diagnoses for this reason. It is also important to remember that it has not been proven that such additional imaging does anything other than to demonstrate more opacified urinary tract segments. It is not clear that any additional pathology will be detected.

OTHER ANCILLARY MANEUVERS

A number of ancillary maneuvers have been added to the CT protocol in an attempt to improve urinary tract distention and opacification, with the hope that resulting improvements would augment sensitivity in detecting urinary tract lesions. These maneuvers have included abdominal compression, saline hydration, and injection of low-dose diuretics. Abdominal compression has been used for CTU due to its long-established acceptance for conventional IVU. Diuretics have been included in MR urography protocols. Research evaluating the efficacy of any of these maneuvers in improving urinary tract visualization is preliminary.

Abdominal Compression Use of compression bands has been advocated by a number of researchers (5,6,12,29).

When CTU is performed with abdominal compression, the bands are usually placed over the patient and tightened when the contrast injection begins. Ideally, an initial set of excretory phase images is obtained of the kidneys and proximal ureters. Then, the compression is released, and the distal ureters are imaged. Thus, if compression is used properly, the excretory phase images are divided into two different components.

Compression bands are inexpensive and easily applied, although their use requires an additional equipment purchase. Also, compression is not popular with technologists because it requires more time and increases the complexity of the CTU protocol.

Three studies have advocated use of compression for excretory phase renal CT or CTU. In the first study, McNicholas and colleagues (29) compared supine compression CTU with supine noncompression and prone noncompression CTU, as well as with IVU with compression. Excretory phase images were obtained at 600 seconds. The authors assigned opacification scores to each renal collecting system and ureter (which was divided into five segments). There was no significant difference between CTU and IVU in opacification of the intrarenal collecting systems and proximal and mid ureters. Among the CTU techniques, supine compression scanning and prone positioning resulted in better opacification scores than did supine noncompression scanning. Compression release scanning produced comparable distal ureteral opacification to IVU but superior opacification to the other CT urographic techniques. The authors concluded that compression CTU is comparable to IVU.

In a second study, Heneghan and associates (12) compared urinary tract opacification obtained during compression and compression release excretory phase images obtained at 180 seconds with that obtained during IVU. They found that CT demonstrated significantly better opacification of the intrarenal collecting systems and mid ureters than did IVU (although the differences in opacification for some segments were minor), and that proximal and distal ureteral opacification was comparable for both studies.

In the third study, Caoili and colleagues (30) observed that more intrarenal collecting system and proximal ureteral urinary tract segments were opacified, and the degree of distention of the opacified segments imaged at 300 seconds was greater (by a mean of approximately 1 mm), when compression was utilized during renal mass CT. This was the first study that considered urinary tract opacification and distention as two different features.

A study has been performed in which a variety of ancillary CTU maneuvers (including compression) were compared to each other and a control group (26). Excretory phase images were obtained at both 300 and 450 seconds. Although patients who were examined with a compression device had better intrarenal collecting system opacification and distention than those who did not, the differences were minor and not significant. The authors concluded that use of compression did not significantly improve urinary tract visualization.

It is difficult to compare the previously discussed studies because there were differences in the CTU protocol as well as the classification systems used to score the urinary tract appearances. However, one common feature of the studies can be identified: Improvement in opacification and distention when compression is used is, at best, only slight.

Saline Hydration A popular ancillary maneuver involves the use of pre- and intraprocedural hydration to maximize urinary excretion and, hence, upper urinary tract distention and opacification. Preprocedural hydration has been performed commonly by administering normal saline intravenously to the patient. This technique was first described by McTavish and associates (7). In this study, 250 ml of (0.9%) normal saline was administered by gravity infusion (not with a power injector) immediately following contrast material injection. The infusion continued until the excretory phase images were obtained at 8 to 10 minutes. Patients placed in supine and prone positions received normal saline hydration during CTU. They were compared to patients who did not receive saline as well as patients undergoing IVU. There were no statistically significant differences in opacification scores in patients examined in the prone position. However, opacification scores for the distal ureters were significantly better when patients received saline hydration. There were no significant differences in opacification scores for the intrarenal collecting system or proximal or lower ureters. The authors concluded that use of saline hydration was effective in improving urinary tract opacification.

In a follow-up study (26), intravenous hydration with 250 ml of normal (0.9%) saline administered intravenously by gravity infusion just prior to the contrast material injection was also found to significantly improve both graded opacification of the intrarenal collecting systems and proximal ureters and subjectively graded study quality of the intrarenal collecting systems. However, there was no significant improvement of intrarenal collecting system or proximal ureteral distention or in opacification or distention of the distal ureters. Although this series demonstrated some advantages to using saline, even the significant differences were minor.

In another study (31), administration of normal saline after completion of the first dose of contrast material injected as part of a split bolus protocol had no effect on urinary tract opacification. Distention of some urinary tract segments did increase slightly when the saline-hydrated patients were compared to a control group. However, the authors utilized only 100 ml of saline, a substantially lower volume than was administered in the other studies.

Sudakoff and colleagues (28) administered 250 ml of normal saline intravenously immediately following infusion of the first bolus of contrast material during split bolus CTU. Urinary tract opacification in each of six different urinary tract segments was assessed using a binary classification system. Each segment was considered either completely opacified or incompletely opacified. Hydration with normal saline did not result in significantly more completely opacified urinary tract segments.

Because each of the previously discussed studies evaluating the benefits of intravenous saline hydration used different CT urography protocols, with differences in contrast media dose, saline volume, and timing, and different analytical methods, it is difficult to draw any firm conclusions. There may be some benefit. Intravenous saline is inexpensive, easy to administer, and well tolerated by nearly all patients. Thus, if one wishes to perform optimal quality CT urograms, use of saline hydration is considered acceptable but not essential.

Oral Hydration Another possible approach is to hydrate patients orally prior to performing CTU. This is a reasonable alternative, although care must be taken to ensure that older patients or patients with a history of congestive heart failure do not ingest too much fluid.

Oral administration of large amounts of fluid appears to be well-tolerated. Kawamoto and colleagues (32) reported results of administering water to 50 patients immediately prior to CTU. In this study, patients were asked to drink 750 to 1000 ml of water within 15 to 20 minutes of CT urography. No other maneuvers were utilized. The authors reported that "nearly all patients" were able to drink this amount of water without difficulty. Subsequently, the CTU studies were analyzed by two reviewers, who found the urinary tract to be completely or nearly completely opacified in the vast majority of patients. Poor opacification (<80%) was noted by each reviewer in 5% and 5% of intrarenal collecting systems, 2% and 2% of renal pelves, 14% and 17% of upper ureters, and 23% and 33% of lower ureters. Although this study did not assess urinary tract distention and did not compare the use of oral hydration with other maneuvers, the authors concluded that an oral hydration-only approach produces acceptable urinary tract opacification during CTU. These results again confirmed that the lower or distal ureter is the most difficult segment to opacify.

Diuretics Diuretics have been used effectively for MR urography. It is not surprising that their use improves visualization of nondistended, nonobstructed urinary tracts on MR urography since they dramatically increase urinary excretion. Another effect of diuretic administration is a decrease in the concentration of excreted contrast material in urine.

These effects would potentially improve urinary tract visualization during CTU, primarily by improving intrarenal collecting system and ureteral distention. Additionally, there might be an increase in the number of opacified urinary tract segments. Finally, by decreasing the concentration of the iodinated contrast material in the urinary tract, it might be easier to detect tiny urothelial abnormalities that might otherwise be obscured.

Not surprisingly, several investigators have advocated administering furosemide when performing CTU (11,33,34). Use of diuretics for CTU was first reported by Nolte-Ernstung et al. (33), who found that when 10 mg of furosemide was administered intravenously 3 to 5 minutes before contrast media was infused, urinary tract opacification was excellent, allowing for near-complete or complete opacification of 32 renal collecting systems and 30 of 32 ureters in 16 patients.

Silverman et al. (34) reported that intravenous administration of 10 mg of furosemide during CTU resulted in significantly better middle and distal ureteral opacification and distention compared to intravenous saline. Interestingly, there was no further improvement in opacification or distention when patients were administered both saline and furosemide. The authors concluded that CTU image quality was best when furosemide was administered alone.

Although it is likely that furosemide administration does improve the overall quality of a CT urogram, its use increases study complexity. At most institutions in the United States, a specific order for its administration must be given. Usually, the injection must be performed by a nurse or physician and not by a technologist. This might slow CT throughput, at least slightly. Complications might occur rarely in patients whose fluid balance is brittle or in patients with allergies. Still, low-dose furosemide is extremely safe and very well tolerated. At one institution, no complications have been encountered in more than 2.5 years of its regular use for CTU (Stuart Silverman, personal communication).

In summary, any of the previously described ancillary maneuvers can be used in a CTU protocol, although it is difficult to assess the effects of each maneuver. It is not clear whether the observed increases in urinary tract distention and opacification have any effect on improving lesion detection.

IMAGE RECONSTRUCTION AND REFORMATTED IMAGES

Many CTU protocols include multiplanar reformatted images or three-dimensional (3D) reconstructions. These images can be created by a radiologist if the study is being interpreted at a workstation with 3D reconstruction and multiplanar reformatting capability. Due to improvements in software, image reformatting is now easily performed, requiring minimal effort and time. An increasing number of institutions rely on specially trained 3D CT technologists to generate these images.

Reformatted images are often preferred by referring physicians because anatomy and pathology can be demonstrated in a fashion similar to that obtained with IVU or to that encountered during surgery. However, to the interpreting radiologist, reformatted images only occasionally add helpful information to the axial images. In fact, the three most common 3D reconstruction techniques, volume rendering and maximum and average intensity projection images created from thick slabs, cannot be used in place of standard axial image review. In a review of 27 urothelial neoplasms, Caoili et al. (9) observed that of the 24 neoplasms that could be retrospectively visualized on axial excretory phase CTU images, only 6 (25%) could be seen on the 3D reconstructed images. In addition, 3D images are limited in their capacity to depict other intra-abdominal organs. Extra-urinary findings have

been found in many patients undergoing CTU when axial images are reviewed (35).

In comparison to the limited utility of 3D reconstructed images, multiplanar reformatted images, when obtained using sufficiently thin collimation, might be able to substitute for the axial images. In a study by Feng and colleagues (36), sensitivity for the detection of urothelial neoplasms was equivalent when 1.25-mm-thick axial images were compared to 1.25-mm-thick coronal reformatted images. Despite reviewer inexperience with coronal image review, the coronal images, which were much fewer in number (averaging just over 100 rather than nearly 600), were evaluated more quickly, resulting in increased throughput.

IMAGE REVIEW

Since a large number of images are created, image review, whether axial, reformatted images, or both, is best performed on a picture archiving and communication system (PACS) workstation. Also, excretory phase images should be reviewed utilizing very wide windows. If this is not done, small urinary tract lesions might be completely obscured by the high attenuation excreted contrast material in the renal collecting systems, ureters, or bladder (14).

OVERVIEW/POSSIBLE RECOMMENDED TECHNIQUES

As the previous discussion has shown, there is no clear consensus on the best way to perform CTU, although an understanding of how the technique can be optimized is beginning to develop. Still, the wide variety of different scanners on which CTU is being performed also makes the situation confusing. A few years ago, only a few 16-row multidetector scanners were available. Now, 64-row multidetector technology is becoming widespread. Techniques currently utilized on 16-row multidetector scanners at two institutions are shown in Tables 2.1 and 2.2 as approaches to CTU that have been found successful.

SUMMARY

The CT urographic technique continues to evolve. Although work is still preliminary, several general principles should be followed. Reliance on combinations of IVU and CT or sole reliance on CT scan projection radiographs for excretory phase imaging is no longer justified. Sensitivity in lesion detection using these approaches is less than that for axial excretory phase image acquisition. Three-phase or two-phase split bolus studies can be successfully performed. Thin section excretory phases should be obtained using a thickness of ≤3 mm between 7.5 and 15 minutes after the injection of contrast material begins. Ancillary maneuvers may be helpful, although the effect of compression

Table 2.1. CT Urography Three-Phase Protocol (Single Bolus)[a]

	University of Michigan Hospital	Brigham and Women's Hospital
Oral preparation	None	900 ml water
CT scout images	Anteroposterior and lateral views	Anteroposterior views
Noncontrast series		
Image thickness	5 mm	5 mm
Reconstruction interval	5 mm	5 mm
Contrast material injection	150 ml of 300 mg I/ml at 3 ml/sec	100 ml of 300 mg I/ml at 3 ml/sec
Nephrographic series		
Delay	100 sec	100 sec
Image thickness	2.5 mm	3 mm
Reconstruction interval	1.25 mm	1.5 mm
Excretory series		
Delay	720 sec (12 min)	900 sec (15 min)
Collimation (for reformatting)	1.25 mm	0.75 mm
Preliminary reconstruction interval (for reformatting)	0.625 mm	0.5 mm
Image thickness (for viewing)	2.5 mm	3 mm
Reconstruction interval (for viewing)	1.25 mm	3 mm
Reformatted images	Coronal average intensity projection 2.5 × 1.25 mm, and AP and bilateral oblique volume rendered images	Coronal 3 × 1.5 mm multiplanar reformatted images, curved reformatted images along each ureter, AP and bilateral oblique volume rendered images, and maximum intensity projection images
Ancillary maneuvers	250 ml 0.9% normal saline IV, wide open gravity infusion, beginning at the time of IV insertion	Furosemide 10 mg IV, 2–3 min prior to contrast material injection. If allergy to furosemide, sulfonamides, systolic blood pressure <90 mm Hg, administer 250 ml of 0.9% (normal) saline IV after the contrast material instead of furosemide

[a]These protocols are written for a 16-channel MDCT scanner.

is, at best, mild. Saline hydration may be helpful. Preliminary data on furosemide administration are promising. It should be stressed, however, that the effect of all the ancillary maneuvers on lesion detection is unknown. Although coronal or sagittal reformatted images may be created that are equally effective as axial images in identifying urinary tract pathology (if images are thin enough), standard 3D reconstructions are insensitive and should serve only as adjuncts to other images. Image review is best accomplished on a PACS workstation and must include evaluation of excretory phase scans utilizing wide windows.

Table 2.2. CT Urography Two-Phase Protocol (Split Bolus)[a]

	University of Michigan Hospital	Brigham and Women's Hospital
Oral preparation	None	900 ml water
Scout images	Anteroposterior and lateral	Anteroposterior
Unenhanced images		
Image thickness	5 mm	3 mm
Reconstruction interval	5 mm	3 mm
First contrast material injection	75 ml 300 mg I/ml at 3 ml/sec	50 ml 300 mg I/ml at 2 ml/sec
Delay	600 sec (10 min)	360 sec (6 min)
Second contrast material injection	100 ml 300 mg I/ml at 3 ml/sec	100 ml 300 mg I/ml at 3 ml/sec
Delay	100 sec	100 sec
Combined nephrographic/ excretory phase series		
Collimation (for reformatting)	1.25 mm	0.75 mm
Reconstruction interval (for reformatting)	0.625 mm	0.5 mm
Image thickness (for viewing)	2.5 mm	3 mm
Reconstruction interval (for reformatting)	1.25 mm	3 mm
Reformatted images	Coronal average intensity projection 2.5 × 1.25 mm, anterior and 30 degree bilateral oblique volume rendered images	Coronal 3 × 1.5 mm multiplanar reformatted images, curved reformatted images along each ureter, AP and bilateral oblique volume rendered images, and maximum intensity projection images
Ancillary maneuvers	250 ml 0.9% normal saline IV, wide open gravity infusion, beginning at the time of IV insertion	Furosemide 10 mg IV, 2–3 min prior to contrast material injection. If allergy to furosemide, sulfonamides, systolic blood pressure <90 mm Hg, administer 250 ml of 0.9% (normal) saline IV after the contrast material instead of furosemide

[a]These protocols are written for a 16-channel MDCT scanner.

REFERENCES

1. Perlman ES, Rosenfield AT, Wexler JS, et al. CT urography in the evaluation of urinary tract disease. *J Comput Assist Tomogr.* 1996;20: 620–626.

2. McCollough CH, Bruesewitz MR, Vrtiska TJ, et al. Image quality and dose comparison among screen-film, computed and CT scanned projection radiography: applications to CT urography. *Radiology.* 2001;221:395–403.

3. Kawashima A, Vrtiska TJ, LeRoy AJ, et al. CT urography. *Radiographics.* 2004;24:S35–S58.

4. Kawashima A, LeRoy AJ, King BF, et al. Comparison of CT scanned projection radiographs (SPR) utilizing enhanced algorithms with original CT scan SPR and conventional screen-film radiographs (FSR) in detecting urolithiasis and with respect to image quality. *Radiology.* 2002;225(P):236.

5. Chow LC, Sommer FG. Multidetector CT urography with abdominal compression and three-dimensional reconstruction. *Am J Roentgenol.* 2001;177:849–855.

6. Caoili EM, Cohan RH, Korobkin M, et al. Urinary tract abnormalities: initial experience with multi-detector row CT urography. *Radiology.* 2002;222:353–360.

7. McTavish JD, Jinzaki M, Zou KH, et al. Multi-detector row CT urography: comparison of strategies for depicting the normal urinary collecting system. *Radiology.* 2002;225:783–790.

8. McCarthy CL, Cowan NC. Multidetector CT urography (MD-CTU) for urothelial imaging. *Radiology.* 2002;225(P):237.

9. Caoili EM, Cohan RH, Inampudi P, et al. MDCT urography of upper tract urothelial neoplasms. *Am J Roentgenol.* 2005;184:1873–1881.

10. Lang EK, Macchia RJ, Thomas R, et al. Computerized tomography tailored for the assessment of microscopic hematuria. *J Urol.* 2002;167:547–554.

11. Cornud F, Bienvenu M, Guerini H, et al. Diagnosis of upper tract transitional cell carcinoma (TCC) with a single phase multi-detector CT urography. Paper presented at the 12th annual meeting of the

European Society of Urogenital Radiology, Ljubljana, Slovenia, September, 2005.

12. Heneghan JP, Kim DH, Leder RA, et al. Compression CT urography: a comparison with IVU in the opacification of the collecting system and ureters. *J Comput Assist Tomogr.* 2001;25:343–347.

13. Mueller-Lisse UG, Meindl T, Coppenrath E, et al. Delineation of upper urinary tract segments at low-dose multidetector CT urography: retrospective comparison with a standard protocol. Paper presented at the 12th annual meeting of the European Society of Urogenital Radiology, Ljubljana, Slovenia, September, 2005.

14. Hilmes MA, Caoili EM, Cohan RH, et al. Evaluation of the ability of multi-detector CT urography and different windowing to detect urinary tract pathology. Paper presented at the 29th scientific assembly of the Society of Uroradiology, Phoenix, AZ, March, 2004.

15. Meindl T, Coppenrath E, Degenhardt C, et al. Retrospective analysis of ureteral distention as function of delay time after IV contrast media injection followed by IV saline infusion in CT-urography. Paper presented at the 12th annual meeting of the European Society of Urogenital Radiology, Ljubljana, Slovenia, September, 2005.

16. Townsend B, Silverman SG, Bhagwat J, et al. Current practice of CT urography by uroradiologists: a survey of the Society of Uroradiology. Paper presented at the 31st scientific assembly of the Society of Uroradiology, Kauai, HI, February, 2006.

17. Chai RY, Jhaveri K, Saini S, et al. Comprehensive evaluation of patients with haematuria on multi-slice computed tomography scanner: protocol design and preliminary observations. *Australas Radiol.* 2001;45:536–538.

18. Kekelidze M, Dijkshoorn ML, Dwarkasing S, et al. Initial experience and perspectives of a low-dose two-phase "triple bolus single scan" multidetector CT urography (MDCTU) protocol. *Eur Radiol.* 2006;16(Suppl):181.

19. Dillman JR, Caoili EM, Cohan RH, et al. Comparison of distention and opacification utilizing three-phase vs. split-bolus two-phase multi-detector row CT urography. Paper presented at the 31st scientific assembly of the Society of Uroradiology, Kauai, HI, February, 2006.

20. Sussman SK, Illescas FF, Opalacz JP, et al. Renal streak artifact during contrast enhanced CT: comparison of high versus low osmolality contrast media. *Abdom Imaging.* 1993;18:180–185.

21. Heneghan JP, McGuire KA, Leder RA, et al. Helical CT for nephrolithiasis and ureterolithiasis: comparison of conventional and reduced radiation-dose techniques. *Radiology.* 2003; 229:575–580.

22. Tack D, Sourtzis S, Delpierre I, et al. Low-dose unenhanced multidetector CT of patients with suspected renal colic. *Am J Roentgenol.* 2003;180:305–311.

23. Degenhart C, Meindl T, Coppenrath E, et al. CT-urography (CTU) in the evaluation of upper urinary tract disease: retrospective comparison of standard-dose and low-dose CTU protocols. *Eur Radiol.* 2006;16(Suppl):180.

24. Kemper J, Regier M, Bansmann M, et al. Low-dose CT urography: image quality analysis during gradual tube current reduction. Animal experience. *Eur Radiol.* 2006;16(Suppl):180.

25. Walter J, Caoili EM, Cohan RH, et al. Can unenhanced scans be eliminated during multi-detector CT urography (MDCTU) without sacrificing study accuracy? Paper presented at the 30th scientific assembly of the Society of Uroradiology, San Antonio, TX, February, 2005.

26. Caoili EM, Inampudi P, Cohan RH, et al. Optimization of multi-detector row CT urography: effect of compression, saline administration, and prolongation of acquisition delay. *Radiology.* 2005;235: 116–123.

27. Sudakoff GS, Guralnick M, Langenstroer P, et al. CT urography of urinary diversions with enhanced CT digital radiography: preliminary experience. *Am J Roentgenol.* 2005;184:131–138.

28. Sudakoff GS, Dunn DP, Hellman RS, et al. Opacification of the genitourinary collecting system during MDCT urography with enhanced CT digital radiography: nonsaline versus saline bolus. *Am J Roentgenol.* 2006;186:122–129.

29. McNicholas MMJ, Raptopoulos VD, Schwartz RK, et al. Excretory phase CT urography for opacification of the urinary collecting system *Am J Roentgenol.* 1998;170:1261–1267.

30. Caoili EM, Cohan RH, Korobkin M, et al. Effectiveness of abdominal compression during helical renal CT. *Acad Radiol.* 2001;8:1100–1106.

31. Maher MM, Jhaveri KS, Lucey BC, et al. Does the administration of saline flush during CT urography (CTU) improve ureteric distention and opacification? A prospective study. *Radiology.* 2001;221(P):500.

32. Kawamoto S, Horton KM, Fishman EK. Opacification of the collecting system and ureters on excretory phase CT using oral water as contrast medium. *Am J Roentgenol.* 2006;186:136–140.

33. Nolte-Ernsting CC, Wildberger JE, Borchers H, et al. Multi-slice CT urography after diuretic injection: initial results. *Rofo Fortschr Geb Rontgenstr Neuen Bildgeb Verfahr.* 2001;173:176–180.

34. Silverman SG, Akbar SA, Mortele KJ, et al. Multi-detector row CT urography: comparison of furosemide and saline as adjuncts to contrast medium for depicting the normal urinary collecting system. *Radiology.* 2006;240:749–755.

35. Liu W, Mortele KJ, Silverman SG. Incidental extraurinary findings at MDCT urography in patients with hematuria: prevalence and impact on imaging costs. *Am J Roentgenol.* 2005;185:1051–1056.

36. Feng F, Caoili EM, Cohan RH, et al. Coronal vs standard axial image review CT urography. Paper presented at the 30th scientific assembly of the Society of Uroradiology, San Antonio, TX, February, 2005.

CHAPTER THREE

RADIATION CONSIDERATIONS

RICHARD D. NAWFEL, MS

STUART G. SILVERMAN, MD

Medical x-rays account for the greatest proportion (58%) of nonnatural (man-made) radiation exposure in the United States (1). With the emergence of multidetector CT, the number of multiple-acquisition CT exams, such as CT urography, has increased substantially (2–7). As a result, the concern for controlling the dose associated with CT has intensified. CT urography is an exam that is being used in many institutions as a replacement for conventional intravenous urography. Whereas conventional urography includes several radiographs of the abdomen and pelvis, CT urography usually consists of multiple CT acquisitions of the abdomen and pelvis (7–10). The dose from CT urography may be considerably higher than that of conventional urography. As the utilization of CT urography becomes widespread, it is important to understand the implication of radiation doses and the associated risks.

Radiation risk, CT dose quantities, factors affecting dose, and means for reducing dose are reviewed. It is hoped that radiologists will use this information when considering appropriateness of CT urography and when developing CT urography imaging protocols.

RADIATION RISK

One of the most significant potential risks to patients who are examined with diagnostic CT is an increased probability of cancer due to the radiation exposure from x-rays. This risk is known as a *stochastic effect*. A stochastic effect is defined as one in which the probability of occurrence, rather than the severity of the effect, is proportional to the radiation dose. Stochastic effects have no threshold dose. In general, radiation doses from diagnostic x-ray imaging exams are considered to be low, and there is still a question as to whether sufficient evidence exists that establishes a risk of cancer at these low doses (11,12). Nevertheless, in clinical practice, current radiation protection standards assume that there is no threshold dose below which the risk of cancer induction is zero. This linear nonthreshold model, substantiated in the report by the Committee on Biological Effects of Ionizing Radiation (1), is used most often in medical applications when considering radiation risk to patients. This model asserts that even the smallest radiation dose poses some finite risk (Fig. 3.1). Conversely, the linear threshold model states that there is a threshold dose below which the risk of cancer induction is zero. Although it is difficult to prove that there is no threshold dose, the linear nonthreshold model is the most conservative one describing radiation risk.

The probability of cancer induction, a stochastic effect defined previously, is the risk associated with x-ray exposure from CT. Conversely, radiation produces nonstochastic effects, or deterministic effects. These are effects in which there is usually an associated threshold. For nonstochastic effects, the severity of the effect is proportional to the radiation dose (13). Examples of nonstochastic effects are erythema and cataract induction. The dose associated with a CT exam is well below the threshold for these nonstochastic effects.

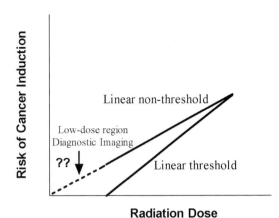

Figure 3.1 Two linear radiation risk models illustrating the relationship between risk of cancer induction and radiation dose.

The radiation risk from a single CT examination is considered small. However, compared to other diagnostic x-ray imaging procedures, the doses patients receive from a single CT exam are higher. There are several reasons for this. Since with CT the x-ray tube rotates around the patient, a CT acquisition delivers more radiation to the patient than a projection radiograph in which the x-ray tube exposes the patient from a single projection. This can lead to a substantially higher dose from CT to a specific region of the body or to critical organs compared to conventional radiography. In addition, many CT protocols, including CT urography, involve multiple acquisitions. This leads to an increased absorbed dose to the patient and thus an increased radiation risk compared to a single CT acquisition. Lastly, CT is being used in medical practice much more frequently than in the past, and CT contributes more medical radiation exposure to the population than any other imaging procedure (14,15).

RADIATION DOSE DESCRIPTORS

The terms *radiation dose* and *absorbed dose* are used to describe the energy absorbed per unit mass of an irradiated material (16). The unit of radiation dose is the gray (Gy). Radiation doses from diagnostic x-ray exams may be expressed in centigray (cGy), milligray (mGy), or microgray (μGy), depending on the magnitude. The older, conventional unit for radiation dose is the rad; 1 Gy = 100 rad. For any x-ray exam, the absorbed dose can be specified for a particular organ of interest, such as skin, thyroid, or bone marrow. Organ doses are usually estimated using radiation output data from the imaging system together with x-ray exposure factors used during the patient exam (17). Patient doses can also be measured during x-ray exams with special dosimeters.

Effective dose, previously called effective dose equivalent, is the dose quantity that accounts for nonuniform irradiation, and it is routinely used to estimate the radiation risk for a CT exam. The effective dose corresponds to the same radiation risk of cancer and genetic effects, whether the radiation is received uniformly by the whole body or nonuniformly, and accounts for both the distribution of radiation and the different radiosensitivities of the organs exposed (16). The unit of effective dose is the sievert (Sv). The unit that preceded the sievert was the rem; 1 Sv = 100 rem. Effective doses from single acquisition CT exams typically range from approximately 1 to 10 mSv. These doses are comparable to the annual dose from natural background radiation, approximately 3 mSv.

Radiation dose from CT exams is estimated using a specific dose descriptor, the computed tomography dose index (CTDI). The CTDI is a measure of the integral dose along a dose profile within a tomographic section that takes into account scatter radiation from adjacent tomographic sections (18–23). The CTDI is estimated from measurements in dosimetry phantoms using a pencil ionization chamber or thermoluminescent dosimeters. CTDI measurements are performed during routine quality assurance dose assessment of a CT scanner. The CTDI concept has been applied to single-slice scanners, including spiral and non-spiral CT; however, with the advent of multidetector CT, the CTDI methodology is limited in estimating dose. Ionization chambers currently used do not measure completely the increased scatter radiation for beam widths associated with multidetector CT scanners. New methods for evaluating radiation dose have been proposed (24–26). There are several dose quantities that have been developed to modify the CTDI concept so that it can be applied to multidetector CT acquisitions. It is important to be aware that there are various CTDI descriptors, and a reported dose should explicitly reflect which CTDI value was measured.

Despite these limitations, CTDI values near the surface and at the central location of a dosimetry phantom can be used to estimate the effective dose for a particular CT scanning protocol. Effective dose accounts for the radiosensitivity of each irradiated organ and its contribution to the total radiation risk. Thus, it allows one to compare the radiation risk from CT with the radiation risk associated with other common diagnostic x-ray exams (Table 3.1).

The effective dose from a single abdominal CT acquisition is associated with a risk of approximately 1 chance in 2,500 (0.04%) of fatal cancer induction. This is extremely low compared to the natural incidence of fatal cancer induction (27), which is in the range of 1 in 6.7 (15%) to 1 in 4 (25%). However, the dose patients receive from several CT exams accumulates quickly, and the radiation risk can be substantial, particularly if an exam consists of multiple acquisitions. In addition, the risk is greater in children since their organs are more radiosensitive than are those of adults (28).

A special consideration for patient radiation risk is the exposure to the unborn fetus. The time period of greatest risk from exposure to the fetus is the first trimester. The risk

Table 3.1. Effective Doses for Common Diagnostic Imaging Exams Compared to Natural Sources of Radiation

Source	Effective Dose	
Diagnostic Imaging[a]	mSv	mrem
Radiography (single film)		
PA chest x-ray	0.02	2
Extremity	0.01	1
Dental, single film	0.10	10
Head/neck	0.20	20
KUB	0.55	55
CT (single acquisition)		
Head CT	1.6	160
Chest CT	6.8	680
Abdomen/pelvis CT	8.5	850
CT (three acquisitions)		
CT urography	15.9	1590
Other (natural)		
Coast-to-coast airplane flight	0.05	5
Annual background radiation	3.0	300

[a]Diagnostic imaging exam data from Brigham and Women's Hospital (2004). Estimates assume average-size adult males.

of teratogenic effects, such as organ malformation, growth retardation, mental retardation, or childhood cancer, has been studied extensively, and quantitative risk estimates with associated dose thresholds have been developed (29). These effects have an increased probability of occurring at a threshold fetal dose in the range of 50 to 100 mGy. Most diagnostic imaging procedures result in fetal doses well below this threshold; however, procedures such as CT urography, which may include multiple CT acquisitions of the pelvis, can result in fetal doses that approach this threshold. For pregnant patients undergoing CT urography, the potential radiation risk to the fetus should be considered when evaluating the health benefit of the procedure. Furthermore, the mother may derive some benefit from the CT urogram, whereas the fetus will not.

FACTORS AFFECTING CT DOSE

CT radiation doses can vary considerably between scanners and between institutions. Clinical CT doses are reported as the dose to standard dosimetry phantoms. However, due to large variations in patient size compared to phantom size, these doses may not estimate accurately the dose delivered to patients during a particular CT exam. A patient's radiation risk from a particular CT exam is proportional to the radiation dose delivered during the exam. This dose will depend on the size of the patient, the type of CT scanner, and the imaging protocol used. CT scanner design factors such as beam geometry and beam quality will have an effect on the magnitude and distribution of radiation dose (20). Focal spot size, focal spot to center of rotation distance, and prepatient collimation will also affect the dose distribution to the patient. These factors may vary by scanner manufacturer. Also, special shaped filtration is sometimes used at the x-ray tube to compensate for beam hardening through tissue that can cause inaccuracies in the reconstruction process and lead to image artifacts. These filters reduce the surface dose to the patient over certain anatomical regions and provide a more homogenous dose distribution.

For any given CT scanner, radiation doses for different exams can also vary considerably. Technical exposure factors that define a particular imaging protocol have an effect on patient dose. Some of the factors, such as x-ray tube potential, x-ray tube current, tube filtration, detector beam width or collimation, pitch, and rotation time, affect patient radiation dose. Imaging protocols can vary appreciably depending on the particular region of the body being scanned, and a particular organ may receive a higher dose from one imaging protocol compared to another. Thus, it is important to know the dose for a given imaging protocol and understand how dose varies with technical exposure parameters.

Patient size is another source of variation in estimating radiation dose. In one study, estimates of effective doses from pediatric CT exams were found to be 50% higher than those of corresponding adult exams (30,31). If the same CT x-ray beam is used to expose both small and large patients, the small patients will receive the larger dose. The attenuation of the x-ray beam is much less in the small patient compared to the large patient. Therefore, in a small patient, as the x-ray tube rotates around the patient, the dose at the midline between entrance and exit in the patient is only slightly less than the entrance dose. The midline dose can be as high 80% of the entrance dose in small patients. In the large patient, however, the midline dose can be reduced by as much as 50% due to much greater attenuation. Other studies have demonstrated that patient size has a large effect on radiation dose in CT (30,31).

CT UROGRAPHY

We determined that at our institution, effective doses from CT urography ranged from approximately 10 to 20 mSv for a particular protocol that consisted of three CT acquisitions (32). The first and last acquisitions included the entire abdomen and pelvis in the exposed volume, whereas the second acquisition included only exposure to the region of the kidneys. The mean effective dose for the entire CT urography exam (14.8 mSv) was approximately 1.5 times the mean effective dose for patients examined with conventional intravenous urography (9.7 mSv) and slightly more than twice the mean effective dose of a single abdominal/pelvic CT acquisition (6.4 mSv). Others have also reported similar doses for multiphase CT exams obtained to evaluate patients with suspected urinary tract disease (2,33).

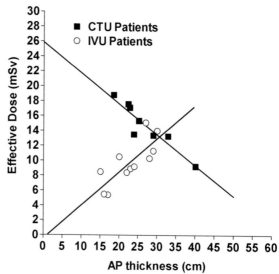

Figure 3.2 Effective dose versus patient thickness for CTU and IVU exams. Effective dose for CTU patients decreased by approximately a factor of two as patient thickness increased by a comparable amount (thickness, 18.5–40 cm), whereas dose for IVU patients increased approximately threefold as patient thickness doubled (15–30 cm). The relation between effective dose and patient size was statistically significant for both CTU ($p = 0.001$) and IVU ($p = 0.004$) exams. This supports the notion of increased radiation risk for smaller patients during CTU, and that technique factors should be adjusted for patient size. From Nawfel RD, Judy PF, Schleipman AR, et al. Patient radiation dose at CT urography and conventional urography. *Radiology*. 2004;232:126–132. Reprinted with permission.

Since radiation dose from CT can vary considerably with patient size, effective dose has been shown to vary in both patients examined with CT urography and patients who received conventional intravenous urography (Fig. 3.2) (32). Of the patients who underwent CT urography, the thinnest patients received an effective dose almost twice that of the larger patients. Results of this study indicated that small adult patients, or pediatric patients, could potentially receive twice the radiation dose and, therefore, twice the radiation risk compared to large patients undergoing CT urography. Considering that CT urography involves exposure to the gonads, there is also concern about the increased radiation risk in pediatric patients because children have a higher radiosensitivity than adults.

DOSE REDUCTION AND FUTURE DEVELOPMENTS

Methods for dose reduction are being developed by CT manufacturers and medical imaging scientists. Reducing dose from CT can be achieved by adjusting technical factors discussed previously that affect dose—that is, tube potential (kVp) or tube current–exposure time product (mAs). For example, assuming all other factors remain constant, decreasing tube potential from 140 to 120 kVp can reduce the patient skin dose by approximately 33%. Similarly, decreasing tube potential from 120 to 80 kVp will reduce skin dose by approximately 70%. Also, decreasing exposure time product will decrease patient dose proportionally. However, decreasing tube potential, tube current, or both increases image noise and may interfere with image quality enough to affect diagnostic accuracy. Usually, an increase in image noise is associated with large patients. To compensate for this degradation in image quality, technologists frequently increase the tube potential and/or tube current from the standard setting in these patients. The result is an improvement in image quality, with the cost of an increased dose to the patient.

Decreasing the overall radiation dose from CT exams could also be accomplished by simply reducing the number of CT acquisitions for a given exam; for example, CT urography could be performed with two acquisitions instead of three (34,35). The mean effective doses for our institution's three-acquisition protocol were, respectively, 6.4 mSv (abdomen and pelvis, unenhanced phase), 2.5 mSv (kidneys, nephrographic phase), and 5.9 mSv (abdomen and pelvis, pyelographic phase) (32). If the nephrographic phase, for example, were eliminated from the protocol, the dose to the patient could be reduced by 17%.

Technology has been developed by manufacturers that can reduce radiation in CT without compromising image quality. Using patient x-ray attenuation information, the CT scanner's x-ray tube current can be modulated at specific locations during the volumetric acquisition (36,37). The attenuation information from anterior–posterior and lateral projection scans is used to program the tube current so that it is adapted to the specific region being scanned. This adaptation takes place both along the patient axis and in the axial plane as the tube is rotating around the patient (38,39). A predefined image quality level is used as a reference level. The scanner software then adjusts the tube current upward or downward from this reference level such that the tube current (and resulting radiation dose) decreases for thin body parts and increases for thick body parts. With this design, unnecessary radiation will be minimized when scanning small patients, and patient doses will be reduced. When scanning large patients, however, radiation dose may increase in order to maintain the predefined image quality level.

CONCLUSION

With any diagnostic imaging exam, the radiation risk to the patient should be considered when compared to the health benefits of the exam. In general, although CT doses are high compared to other diagnostic x-ray exposures, the radiation risk from a single CT acquisition is considered low. As is the case for the number of films during conventional radiography, CT patient dose is proportional to the number of CT acquisitions. Since CT doses are cumulative, radiologists should be aware of this fact when designing protocols for CT urography.

Exposure technique factors should be adjusted during CT exams so that only a sufficient radiation dose is used. Tube potential, tube current, scan pitch, or scan length can all be adjusted, either manually by technologists or using automated methods, to reduce the radiation dose a patient receives during CT urography.

The level of radiation dose used to create images greatly affects image quality. The goal is to use the least amount of radiation that will provide adequate image quality. In general, higher radiation doses provide better image quality, all else being equal. It is the responsibility of the radiologist to determine appropriate scanning technique factors that provide a balance between image quality and radiation dose. A lower dose version of a CT urography protocol might be considered for young patients (e.g., pediatric age groups) when radiation dose is a concern. This could include reducing the number of acquisitions, reducing the volume scanned, or both. Reducing dose to the patient by decreasing technique factors is accompanied by an increase in image noise, and provided that this noise level is tolerable, patient doses can and should be reduced as much as possible.

CT urography provides radiologists with extremely useful, detailed information when imaging the kidneys and urinary tract. However, when choosing among imaging tests, the diagnostic information gained from CT urography should outweigh the radiation risk to the patient.

REFERENCES

1. National Research Council, Committee to Assess Health Risks from Exposure to Low Levels of Ionizing Radiation. *Health risks from exposure to low levels of ionizing radiation, BEIR VII—Phase 2*. Washington, DC: National Academies Press, 2005.

2. Spielmann AL, Heneghan JP, Lee LJ, et al. Decreasing the radiation dose for renal stone CT: a feasibility study of single- and multidetector CT. *Am J Roentgenol*. 2002;178:1058–1062.

3. Nickoloff EL, Alderson PO. Radiation exposures to patients from CT: reality, public perception and policy. *Am J Roentgenol*. 2001;177: 285–287.

4. Brenner D, Elliston C, Hall E, et al. Estimated risks of radiation-induced fatal cancer from pediatric CT. *Am J Roentgenol*. 2001;176:289–296.

5. Slovis TL. CT and computed radiography: the pictures are great, but is the radiation dose greater than required? *Am J Roentgenol*. 2002; 179:39–41.

6. Kalra MK, Prasad S, Saini S, et al. Clinical comparison of standard-dose and 50% reduced-dose abdominal CT: effect on image quality. *Am J Roentgenol*. 2002;179:1101–1106.

7. Frush DP, Slack CC, Hollingsworth CL, et al. Computer-simulated radiation dose reduction for abdominal multidetector CT of pediatric patients. *Am J Roentgenol*. 2002;179:1107–1113.

8. Caoili EM, Cohan RH, Korobkin M, et al. Urinary tract abnormalities: initial experience with multi-detector row CT urography. *Radiology*. 2002;222:353–360.

9. McNicholas MM, Raptopoulos VD, Schwartz RK, et al. Excretory phase CT urography for opacification of the urinary collecting system. *Am J Roentgenol*. 1998;170:1261–1267.

10. McTavish JD, Jinzaki M, Zou KH, et al. Multi-detector row CT urography: comparison of strategies for depicting the normal urinary collecting system. *Radiology*. 2002;225:783–790.

11. Becker K. Threshold or no threshold, that is the question [Editorial]. *Radiat Prot Dosimetry.* 1997;71:3–5.

12. Cohen BL. Cancer risk from low level radiation. *Am J Roentgenol.* 2002;179:1137–1143.

13. National Council on Radiation Protection and Measurements. *Recommendations on limits for exposure to ionizing radiation.* NCRP report no. 91. Bethesda, MD: National Council on Radiation Protection and Measurements, June 1, 1987.

14. Mettler FA Jr, Wiest PW, Locken JA, et al. CT scanning: patterns of use and dose. *J Radiol Prot.* 2000;20(4):347–348.

15. Kalra MK, Maher MM, Toth TL, et al. Strategies for CT radiation dose optimization. *Radiology.* 2004;230:619–628.

16. Alpern EL. *Radiation biophysics.* San Diego: Academic Press; 1998.

17. Wolbarst AB. *Physics of radiology.* Madison, WI: Medical Physics Publishing; 2005.

18. *Federal Register* 481 (1990) (codified at 21 CFR §1020.33). Food and drugs: performance standards for ionizing radiation emitting products-computed tomography (CT) equipment.

19. American Association of Physicists in Medicine. *Specification and acceptance testing of computed tomography scanners*, report no. 39. New York: American Institute of Physics; 1993;52–55.

20. Rothenberg LN, Pentlow KS. CT dose assessment. In: Seibert JA, Barnes GT, Gould RG, eds. *Specification, acceptance testing, and quality control of diagnostic x-ray imaging equipment*, Medical Physics Monograph no. 20. Woodbury, NY: American Institute of Physics; 1994;899–936.

21. Atherton JV, Huda W. CT doses in cylindrical phantoms. *Phys Med Biol.* 1995;40:891–911.

22. Jansen JM, Geleijins J, Zweers D, et al. Calculation of computed tomography dose index to effective dose conversion factors based on measurement of the dose profile along the fan shaped beam. *Br J Radiol.* 1996;69:33–41.

23. Geleijins J, Van Unnik JG, Zoetelief J, et al. Comparison of two methods for assessing patient dose from computed tomography. *Br J Radiol.* 1994;67:360–365.

24. McCollough CH, Zink FE. Performance evaluation of a multi-slice CT system. *Med Phys.* 1999;2223–2230.

25. Dixon RL. A new look at CT dose measurement: beyond CTDI. *Med Phys.* 2003;30:1272–1280.

26. Brenner DJ. Is it time to retire the CTDI for quality assurance and dose optimization? [Letter to the Editor]. *Med Phys.* 2005; 3225–3226.

27. International Commission on Radiological Protection. 1990 Recommendation of the International Commission on Radiological Protection, ICRP Publication 60. *Ann ICRP.* 1991;21(1–3).

28. National Council on Radiation Protection and Measurements. *Risk estimates for radiation protection, recommendations of the National Council on Radiation Protection and Measurements*, NCRP report no. 115. Bethesda, MD: National Council on Radiation Protection and Measurements, December 31, 1993.

29. United Nations Scientific Committee on the Effects of Atomic Radiation. *Genetic and somatic effects of ionizing radiation*, Report to the General Assembly, with annexes. New York: United Nations; 1986.

30. Ware DE, Huda W, Mergo PJ, et al. Radiation effective doses to patients undergoing abdominal CT examinations. *Radiology.* 1999;210:645–650.

31. Huda W, Atherton JV, Ware DE, et al. An approach for the estimation of effective radiation dose at CT in pediatric patients. *Radiology.* 1997;203:417–422.

32. Nawfel RD, Judy PF, Schleipman AR, et al. Patient radiation dose at CT urography and conventional urography. *Radiology.* 2004;232: 126–132.

33. Liu W, Esler SJ, Kenny BJ, et al. Low-dose nonenhanced helical CT of renal colic: assessment of ureteric stone detection and measurement of effective dose equivalent. *Radiology.* 2000;215:51–54.

34. Chow LC, Sommer FG. Multidetector CT urography with abdominal compression and three-dimensional reconstruction. *Am J Roentgenol.* 2001;177(4):849–855.

35. Sudakoff GS, Dunn DP, Hellman RS, et al. Opacification of the genitourinary collecting system during MDCT urography with enhanced CT digital radiography: nonsaline versus saline bolus. *Am J Roentgenol.* 2006;186(1):122–129.

36. Kalender WA, Wolf H, Suess C, et al. Dose reduction in CT by on-line tube current control: principles and validation on phantoms and cadavers. *Eur Radiol.* 1999;9:323–328.

37. Gies M, Suess C, Wolf H, et al. Dose reduction in CT by anatomically adapted tube current modulation: I. Simulation studies. *Med Phys.* 1999;26(11):2235–2247.

38. Kalra MK, Rizzo S, Maher M, et al. Chest CT performed with z-axis modulation: scanning protocol and radiation dose. *Radiology.* 2005;237:303–308.

39. Mulkens TH, Bellinck P, Baeyaert M, et al. Use of an automatic exposure control mechanism for dose optimization in multi-detector row CT examinations: clinical evaluation. *Radiology.* 2005; 237:213–223.

CHAPTER FOUR

NORMAL ANATOMY AND VARIANTS

SUSAN HILTON, MD

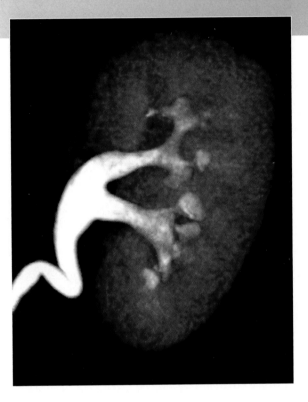

CASE 4-1

History: 41-year-old male with hematuria.

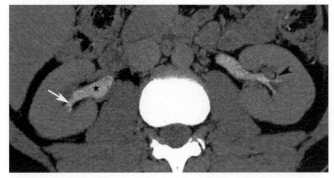

Figure 4.1   A

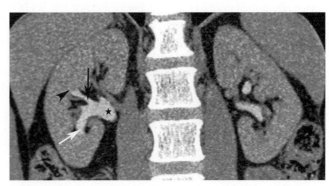

Figure 4.1   B

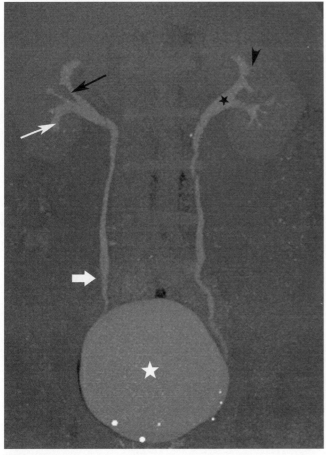

Figure 4.1   C

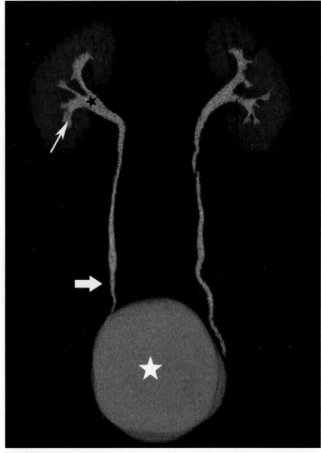

Figure 4.1   D

Findings: Axial image (A), coronal image (B), maximum intensity projection image (C), and volume-rendered image (D) from a normal CT urogram (See Color Fig. 4.1D.). The patient was also administered 10 mg of furosemide intravenously. The renal parenchyma, shown on the volume-rendered image in red, is normal in thickness. The calyces (white arrows) and fornices (black arrowheads) are normal. Other normal structures depicted include the infundibula (black arrows), renal pelves (black stars), ureters (thick white arrow), and bladder (white stars).

Diagnosis: Normal CT urogram

Discussion: The kidneys are retroperitoneal structures located within Gerota's fascia. The superior one-third of the kidney is referred to as the upper pole, the middle one-third as the interpolar region, and the inferior one-third as the lower pole. The kidney is made up of lobes consisting of medullary pyramids that contain the collecting tubules and are surrounded by cortex except at the apex of the pyramids, at the papillae. Each papilla, the innermost portion of the medulla, projects into a calyx. The sharp-edged portion of each calyx extending around the papilla is called the calyceal fornix. The calyces join to form infundibula, which drain into the renal pelvis. Simple calyces are sharp and cup-shaped and drain one renal lobe; compound calyces, more common at the poles of the kidney, are complex in shape and drain several renal lobes (see Case 4-4). The renal pelvis is triangular, with its base in the renal sinus. The apex of the renal pelvis extends inferiorly to join the superior portion of the ureter and form the uretero-pelvic junction. The ureters course inferiorly in the retroperitoneum, anterior to the psoas muscle, and cross the pelvic brim to enter the pelvis. The ureters then enter the bladder at an oblique angle to form the ureterovesical junction. (Case courtesy of Stuart G. Silverman, MD, Brigham and Women's Hospital, Boston, MA.)

History: 46-year-old female with hematuria.

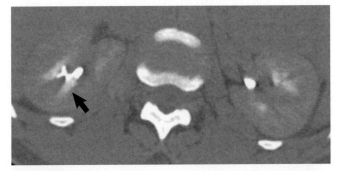

Figure 4.2   A

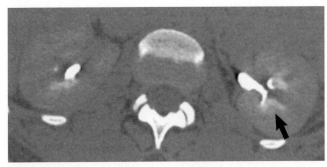

Figure 4.2   B

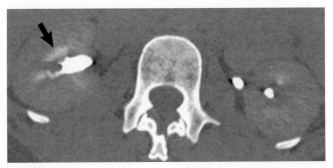

Figure 4.2   C

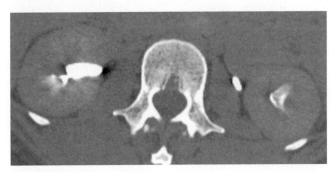

Figure 4.2   D

Findings: Excretory phase axial images (A–D) demonstrate dense radially arranged indistinct opacities in the renal papillae bilaterally (arrows).

Diagnosis: Normal papillary blush

Discussion: In healthy patients undergoing CT urography, visualization of indistinct opacities in the renal pyramids may be seen. This finding has been recognized on intravenous urograms for many years and is thought to be due to the normal concentration of contrast material in the medulla (see Case 11-12). The finding has been reported to be accentuated with low-osmolality contrast media because with the less hyperosmolar low-osmolality contrast media (compared to high-osmolality contrast agents) less fluid is excreted into the tubular lumen and, therefore, the concentration of contrast material is higher than with high-osmolality contrast material. Due to the superior contrast resolution of CT urography compared to intravenous urography, a normal papillary blush is displayed more frequently and more prominently. The "blushlike" appearance should be differentiated from the "brushlike" appearance of multiple, discrete, linear, papillary densities found in renal tubular ectasia (see Cases 4-10, 8-1, and 11-2).

History: 55-year-old female with hematuria.

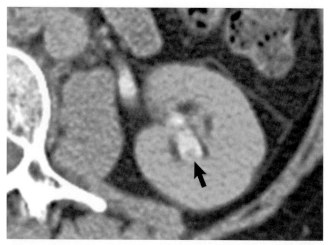

Figure 4.3   A

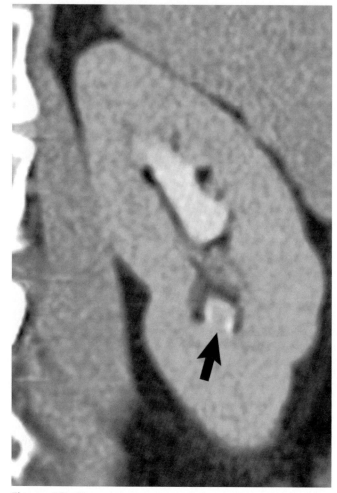

Figure 4.3   B

Findings: Axial (A) and coronal (B) images during the excretory phase of a CT urogram demonstrate an apparent small (4 mm) intraluminal filling defect (arrows) within a calyx of the lower pole of the left kidney.

Diagnosis: Prominent normal papilla

Discussion: CT urography may be used to differentiate a prominent normal papilla from a calyceal-filling defect due to a pathologic process. A prominent normal papilla has a central location within the surrounding calyx, a conical shape, and a smooth contour, as seen in this case (see Case 11-8). Also, in most instances, multiple papillae in the same kidney have the same appearance. Often, the diagnosis can be confirmed by viewing the collecting system in orthogonal planes. (Case courtesy of Stuart G. Silverman, MD, Brigham and Women's Hospital, Boston, MA.)

History: 56-year-old female with hematuria.

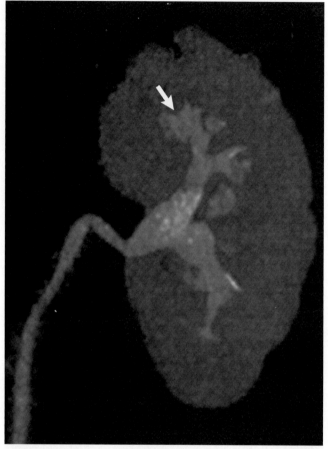

Figure 4.4 A

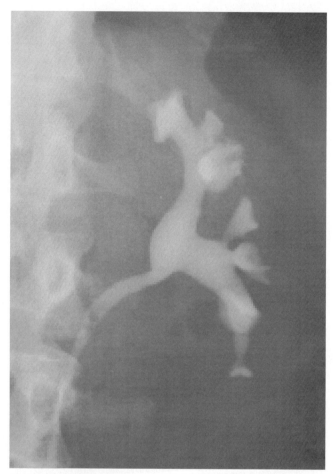

Figure 4.4 B

Findings: A compound calyx of the upper pole of the left kidney (arrow) is displayed on a volume-rendered coronal image of the left kidney (A) and on a left retrograde pyelogram (B).

Diagnosis: Compound calyx

Discussion: Embryologically, the kidney consists of multiple lobes. The collecting ducts of a renal lobe drain through the papilla of a medullary pyramid into a calyx. With simple calyces, each minor calyx empties into a single papilla, such that the number of calyces would equal the number of lobes if all calyces were simple. With compound calyces, multiple papillae empty into a single calyx. Compound calyces are most common in the upper pole and least common in the interpolar region of the kidney. Seventy percent of patients have one or more compound calyces. A compound calyx has also been referred to as a "T shaped" or "hammerhead" calyx. (Case courtesy of Stuart G. Silverman, MD, Brigham and Women's Hospital, Boston, MA.)

History: 77-year-old male with hematuria status post prostatectomy.

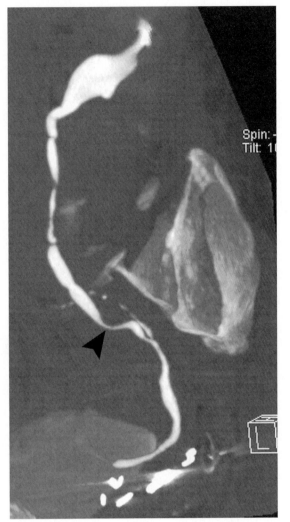

Figure 4.5   A

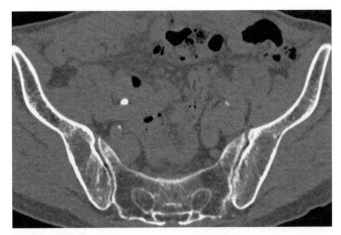

Figure 4.5   B

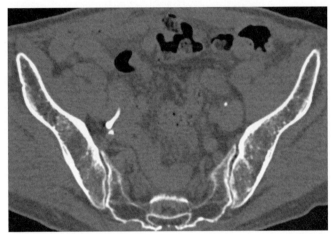

Figure 4.5   C

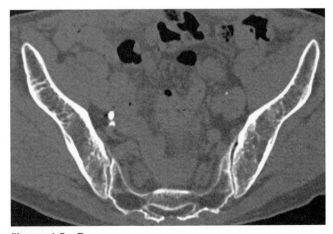

Figure 4.5   D

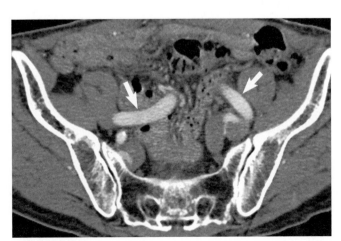

Figure 4.5   E

Findings: Curved planar reconstructed image (A), and axial images (B–D), during the excretory phase shows a narrowed right ureter (arrowhead). Axial image (E) during the arterial phase shows tortuous common iliac arteries (arrows). The ureter is narrowed at the same level as the calcified iliac artery (arrowhead). The right ureter just above the level of the iliac artery is of normal caliber (B), the ureter smoothly narrows as it crosses the tortuous artery (C), and the ureter resumes normal caliber just below the vessel (D).

Diagnosis: Narrowed right ureter due to adjacent atherosclerotic iliac artery

Discussion: The normal ureter is narrowed typically at three sites: the ureteropelvic junction, the point where the ureter crosses the common iliac vessels, and the ureterovesical junction. Narrowing and external impression of the ureter is more pronounced in the presence of atherosclerosis that causes ectasia and tortuosity of the iliac vessels. Vascular impressions may also be seen in the renal pelvis, where a normal, crossing renal artery branch may produce a bandlike or notchlike impression. Prior to the use of CT, this finding on IV urography was occasionally so problematic that angiography was needed to confirm the diagnosis. Today, vascular impressions on the urinary tract can be assessed fully with CT urography.

History: 77-year-old male with hematuria.

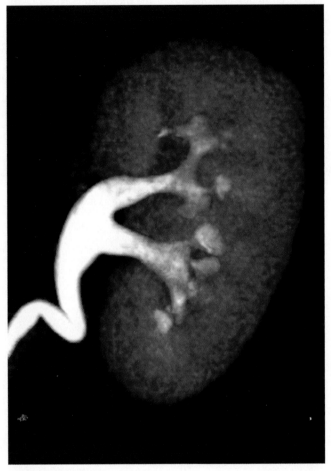

Figure 4.6

Findings: Volume-rendered coronal image from a CT urogram demonstrates a bifid, left-sided, renal collecting system.

Diagnosis: Bifid renal collecting system

Discussion: Duplication anomalies result from the development of a second ureteric bud (complete duplications) or redundant duplication of a single ureteric bud (bifid system). They are the most common congenital anomaly of the urinary tract and are found in 10% of the population. In this patient, two separate renal collecting system components merge to form a single renal pelvis and ureter.

CASE 4-7

History: 92-year-old female with history of bladder cancer.

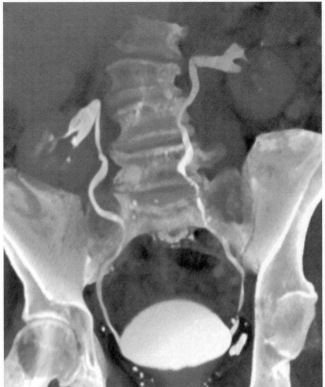

Figure 4.7   A

Figure 4.7   B

Findings: Volume-rendered coronal image (A) and axial image (B) during the excretory phase of a CT urogram demonstrate a low-lying right kidney. The kidney is also abnormally rotated, such that its axis is more horizontal than normally noted. This abnormal rotation accounts for its foreshortened appearance on the coronal image.

Diagnosis: Ptotic right kidney

Discussion: The right renal pelvis is usually located at the level of the L2 vertebra. A ptotic kidney is one that is posi-

tioned inferior to most kidneys. The ureter and renal artery arise from their normal sites. In contrast, an ectopic kidney has a short ureter and an arterial supply that arises ectopically, usually from a major artery in the same vicinity as the ectopic kidney. CT urography is useful to confirm that a kidney that is in an unusual position is not displaced by an adjacent mass.

History: 40-year-old male with hematuria.

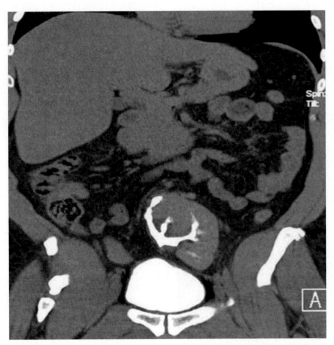

Figure 4.8

Findings: Coronal image during excretory phase of a CT urogram demonstrates a kidney in the left side of the pelvis.

Diagnosis: Left pelvic kidney

Discussion: Pelvic kidneys may be unilateral, bilateral and fused, or solitary. The left kidney is involved in approximately 70% of cases. Four other anomalies are commonly associated with pelvic kidneys: anomalies of rotation, a ureter that inserts high in the renal pelvis, an ectopic ureter, and extrarenal calyces. In this case, the upper pole calyces are extrarenal. Although the pelvic kidney is easily identified on images obtained at CT urography, a pelvic kidney and its collecting system are not always well-evaluated with images obtained using intravenous urography, in which they may be obscured by the overlying sacrum. (Case courtesy of Stuart G. Silverman, MD, Brigham and Women's Hospital, Boston, MA.)

History: 48-year-old male with hematuria.

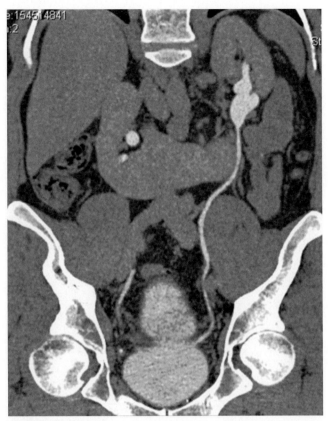

Figure 4.9 A

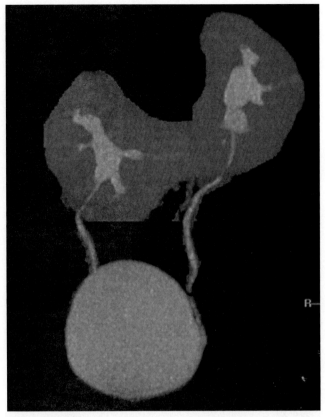

Figure 4.9 B

Findings: Curved planar (A) and maximum intensity projection (B) images during the excretory phase of a CT urogram demonstrate a horseshoe kidney.

Diagnosis: Horseshoe kidney

Discussion: Horseshoe kidney is a common fusion anomaly, occurring in approximately 1 in 400 people (see Case 8-10). Two portions of the kidney are connected by an isthmus consisting of either normal renal tissue or connective tissue. The midline connection develops as the result of fusion of the two metanephrogenic blastemas during embryologic development. The blood supply usually involves multiple arteries from the aorta, iliac arteries, or inferior mesenteric artery. When renal or aortic surgery is planned, CT urography coupled with arterial phase scanning is a useful tool for demonstrating the complex vascular and urinary tract anatomy encountered with this anomaly. (Case courtesy of Stuart G. Silverman, MD, Brigham and Women's Hospital, Boston, MA.)

History: 57-year-old female with recurrent urinary tract infections and suspected right-sided pyelonephritis.

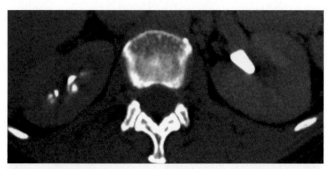

Figure 4.10 A

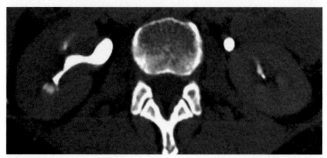

Figure 4.10 B

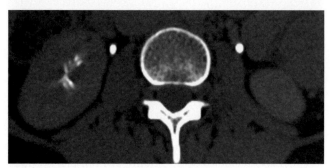

Figure 4.10 C

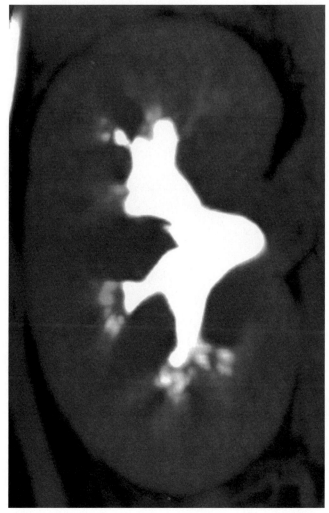

Figure 4.10 D

Findings: Axial (A–C) and oblique coronal maximum intensity projection (D) images from a CT urogram demonstrate discrete linear opacities in the papillae of the right kidney.

Diagnosis: Benign renal tubular ectasia

Discussion: In benign tubular ectasia, the collecting ducts are dilated, measuring more than 0.2 to 0.3 mm in diameter. Because of this, they are typically visible on CT urography as discrete tubular structures, which produce a brushlike appearance in one or more papillae (see Case 11-2). In medullary sponge kidney, the dilated collecting tubules frequently contain calculi. Some authors consider benign tubular ectasia to be the least severe form of medullary sponge kidney, but the definition and diagnostic criteria for medullary sponge kidney are controversial (see Case 8-1). The unenhanced images obtained at CT urography are effective in determining whether there is any associated nephrolithiasis or nephrocalcinosis in patients who have benign renal tubular ectasia identified on the excretory phase series.

CASE 4-11

History: 55-year-old male with hematuria.

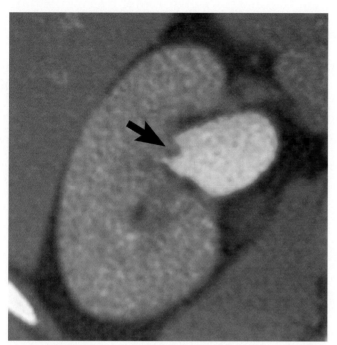

Figure 4.11   A

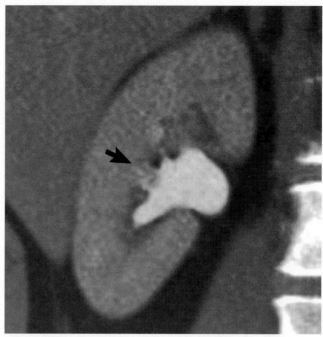

Figure 4.11   B

Findings: Axial (A) and coronal (B) images during the excretory phase of a CT urogram demonstrate a centrally located, conical filling defect (arrows) that projects into the lumen of an infundibulum, at the interpolar region of the right renal kidney.

Diagnosis: Aberrant papilla, arising from the renal pelvis

Discussion: An aberrant papilla is an otherwise normal renal papilla that projects directly into the lumen of an infundibulum or renal pelvis without the presence of a normal, flared minor calyx. Its attachment to one wall is broad, which in this case is seen at CT urography in two planes. It has been postulated that this entity represents direct formation of collecting tubules from the renal pelvis without the development of an intervening calyx. (Case courtesy of Stuart G. Silverman, MD, Brigham and Women's Hospital, Boston, MA.)

History: 48-year-old female with left flank pain.

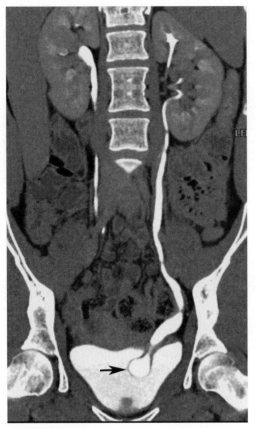

Figure 4.12   A

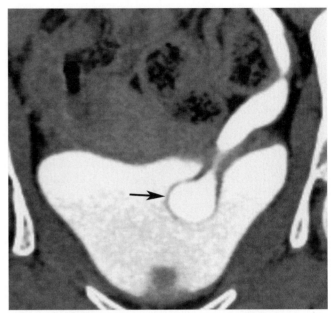

Figure 4.12   B

Findings: Curved planar reformatted image (A) and a magnified view of the curved planar reformatted image (B) demonstrate focal bulbous dilatation of the distal end of the left ureter that is filled with contrast material and protrudes into the contrast material-filled urinary bladder. There is a thin, soft tissue rim outlining the lumen of the distal ureter (arrow). There is mild dilatation of the left ureter just proximal to the ureterocele.

Diagnosis: Small orthotopic (simple) ureterocele

Discussion: A ureterocele is a ballooning of the distal end of the ureter. This appearance of the ureterocele has been called the "cobra-head sign." Ureteroceles may occur with single or duplex ureters. There are two types of ureteroceles—orthotopic and ectopic. With an orthotopic ureterocele, as in this case, the orifice of the ureter and the ureterocele are intravesical (see Case 10-15). With an ectopic ureterocele, the ureterocele lies in the submucosa of the bladder and some part of the ureterocele extends into the bladder neck or urethra. Ureteroceles result from a defect in the development of mesoblast from which the muscle in the ureter and bladder develop. Orthotopic ureteroceles contain an orifice that opens in the normal zone but that is stenotic. Most orthotopic ureteroceles are incidental findings. However, when large, orthotopic ureteroceles may obstruct the bladder neck or cause hydronephrosis. The incidence of stones, persistent infections, and milk of calcium is increased with both types of ureteroceles. (Case courtesy of Stuart G. Silverman, MD, Brigham and Women's Hospital, Boston, MA.)

CASE 4-13

History: 43-year-old female with hematuria.

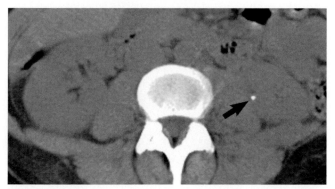

Figure 4.13 A

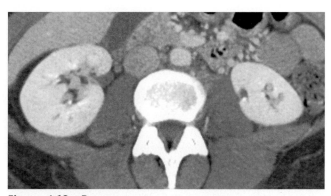

Figure 4.13 B

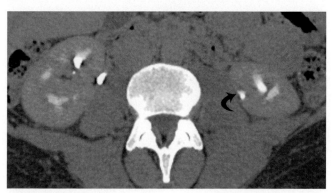

Figure 4.13 C

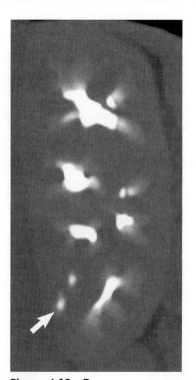

Figure 4.13 D

Findings: Axial unenhanced image (A) demonstrates a small calculus (black arrow) within a fluid-filled structure located medially in the lower pole of the left kidney. Axial images through the same region during the nephrographic (B) and excretory (C) phases demonstrate excreted contrast material layering in the posterior portion of this structure (curved arrow) on the excretory phase image. Coronal maximum intensity projection image during the excretory phase (D) demonstrates the calculus (white arrow) in the inferomedial aspect of the kidney.

Diagnosis: Small calyceal diverticulum containing a tiny calculus

Discussion: Calyceal diverticulum is a rare congenital abnormality in which a urine-filled cavity is connected to a renal calyx, at the fornix, by a narrow isthmus (see Case 8-4). On excretory phase images obtained during CT urography, the diverticulum fills with contrast material via this connection in most cases. This abnormality is believed to result from failure of one of the last generations of tubules to divide and expand normally. Instead of forming an infundibulum of a minor calyx, this tubule becomes a diverticulum. Complications of this entity include infection and stone formation and, rarely, malignancy, rupture, xanthogranulomatous pyelonephritis, or renal abscess.

History: 45-year-old female with voiding dysfunction and a known bladder calculus.

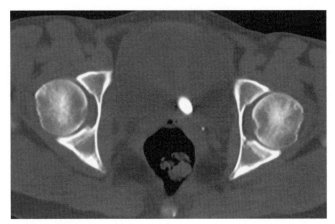

Figure 4.14   A

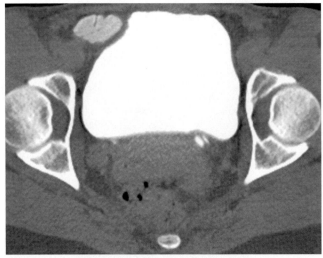

Figure 4.14   C

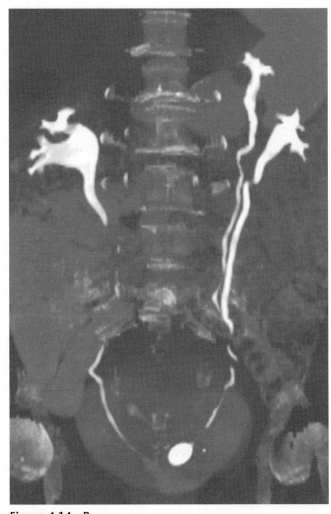

Figure 4.14   B

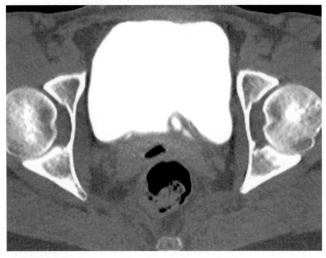

Figure 4.14   D

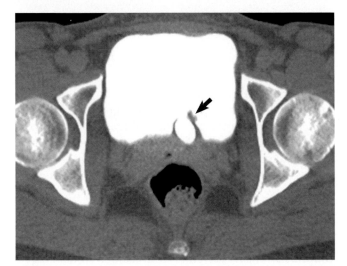

Figure 4.14   E

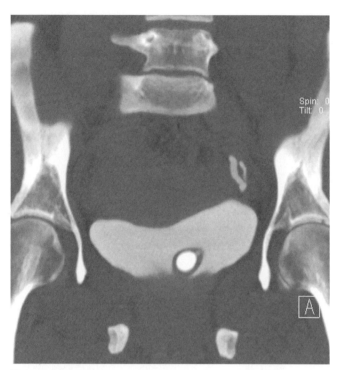

Figure 4.14   F

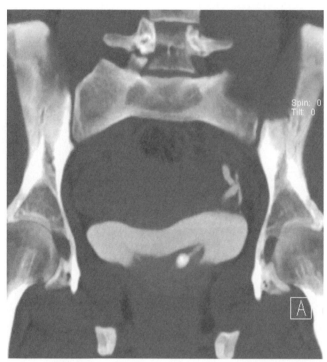

Figure 4.14   G

Findings: Axial, unenhanced image of the urinary bladder (A) demonstrates an ovoid calculus projecting into the posterior aspect of the left side of the urinary bladder. Excretory phase coronal maximum intensity projection image (B) demonstrates a duplicated collecting system on the left side, with two ureters. Axial images (C–E) demonstrate the two left ureters inserting separately into the bladder. The upper pole ureter inserts into a smooth-walled structure containing the calculus. Coronal images (F and G) demonstrate the upper pole ureter entering the calculus-containing ureterocele. A bilobed soft tissue excrescence (arrow) projects from the ureterocele (E).

Diagnosis: Complete duplication of the left collecting system; left-sided ureterocele containing a calculus and adherent inflammatory tissue

Discussion: Ureteroceles may occur at the distal end of single or double ureters. When a ureterocele occurs at the end of a duplicated ureter, it arises most frequently from the ureter draining the upper pole of the kidney, as in this case. Ureteroceles of duplicated ureters that have persisted into adulthood before being discovered are generally smaller than those detected in infants and children. Calculi can form in ureteroceles due to stasis of urine, especially ureteroceles larger than 2 cm in diameter. Intravesical ureteroceles are often detected on intravenous urography in adults. A ureterocele should be differentiated from a pseudo-ureterocele, which refers to dilatation of the distal ureter due to surrounding soft tissue that develops as a result of underlying disease, such as tumor or an impacted calculus. The wall of the ureterocele should be uniform, smooth, and no thicker than 2 mm, whereas the rim of a pseudo-ureterocele is often asymmetric and thick. Multiplanar reconstructions enabled by CT urography allow depiction of the anatomy of the intravesical portions of the normal ureters as well as the walls of ureteroceles.

History: 45 year-old male with hematuria.

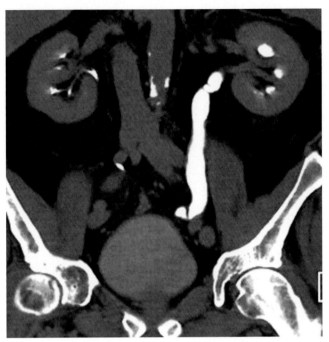

Figure 4.15   A

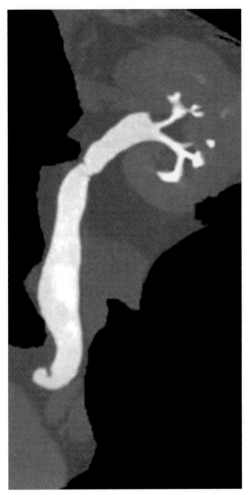

Figure 4.15   B

Findings: Coronal (A) and maximum intensity projection (B) images during the excretory phase of a CT urogram demonstrate a diffusely dilated left ureter above the juxtavesical level, without hydronephrosis.

Diagnosis: Primary megaureter

Discussion: Megaureter is defined as a ureter whose fixed width exceeds 10 mm. Patients with primary megaureter have an abnormally dilated ureter without evidence of significant reflux or anatomic obstruction (see Case 9-22). In this congenital anomaly, there is aperistalsis of the juxtavesical segment of the ureter. The ureter is always dilated above the relatively narrow juxtavesical segment. The cause of the aperistalsis is unclear. Primary megaureter is common in children, but it is also seen in adults. It is more common in males, and there is a left-sided predominance. Primary megaureter can be distinguished from ureteral obstruction due to acquired causes, where dilatation of the intrarenal collecting system also usually present. (Case courtesy of Stuart G. Silverman, MD, Brigham and Women's Hospital, Boston, MA.)

History: 35-year-old female with renal insufficiency.

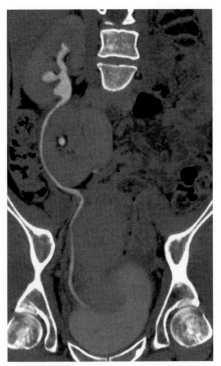

Figure 4.16   A

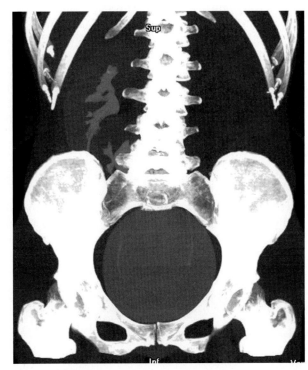

Figure 4.16   B

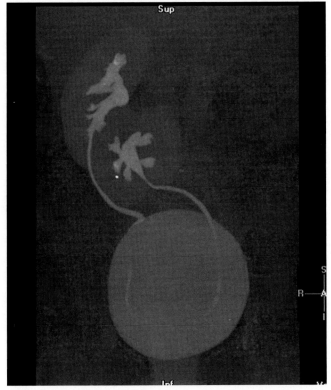

Figure 4.16   C

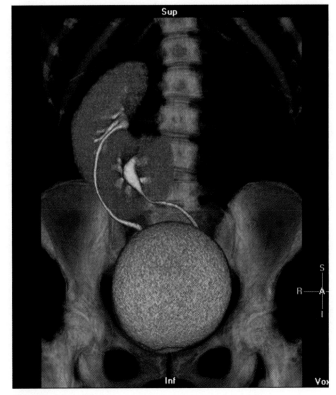

Figure 4.16   D

Findings: Curved planar reformatted image (A), maximum intensity projection image with bone included (B), maximum intensity projection image with bone subtracted (C), and volume-rendered image (D) from a CT urogram demonstrate that the right kidney is in the normal position (See Color Fig. 4.16 D.). The left kidney is on the right side of the abdomen and fused to the inferior pole of the right kidney. The right ureter courses along the lateral margin of the right kidney before taking a normal course into the pelvis. The left ureter crosses from right to left before inserting normally into the left side of the bladder.

Diagnosis: Crossed fused renal ectopia

Discussion: Crossed fused ectopia is a congenital anomaly that occurs when the kidney completely or almost completely crosses the midline to the opposite side of the body and fuses with the contralateral kidney (see Case 8-9). The ureters insert in their normal positions. The ureter from the crossed kidney, therefore, extends across the midline to enter the bladder on the side opposite the fused kidney, as in this case. This anomaly occurs more frequently in males and the fused kidney is found two or three times more often on the right. There are many variations of the pattern of renal parenchymal fusion, including superior ectopia, S-shaped kidney, unilateral lump kidney, unilateral L-shaped kidney, unilateral disc kidney, and inferior ectopia, as in this case. An anomalous blood supply arising from nearby vessels feeds the crossed fused ectopic kidney. Complications include high insertion of the ureter into the renal pelvis that results in an increased incidence of ureteropelvic junction obstruction. Stones may also occur. Associated anomalies include vesicoureteral reflux, unilateral or bilateral duplication, megaureter, renal dysplasia, retrocaval ureter, esophageal atresia, rectovaginal fistula, and omphalocele. (Case courtesy of Stuart G. Silverman, MD, Brigham and Women's Hospital, Boston, MA.)

SUGGESTED READINGS

1. Hodson CJ. The lobar structure of the kidney. *Br J Urol*. 1972;44: 246–261.

2. Bigognari LR, Patel SK, et al. Medullary rays: visualization during excretory urography. *Am J Roentgenol*. 1975;125:795–803.

3. Ohlson L. Normal collecting ducts: visualization at urography. *Radiology*. 1989;170:33–37.

4. Goldstein HM, Reuter SR, Wallace S. Pseudotumor of the renal pelvis caused by arterial impression. *J Urol*. 1974;111(6):735–737.

5. Lefleur RS, Ambos MA, Rothberg M. An unusual vascular impression on the renal pelvis. *Urol Radiol*. 1979;1:117–118.

6. Zagoria RJ. The kidney and retroperitoneum: anatomy and congenital abnormalities. In: Zagoria RJ, ed. *The requisites: genitourinary radiology*. 2nd ed. Philadelphia: Mosby; 2004:51–79.

7. Nino-Murcia M, DeVries PA, Friedland GW. Congenital anomalies of the kidney. In: Pollack HM, McClennan BL, eds. *Clinical urology*. 2nd ed. Philadelphia: Saunders; 2000:690–763.

8. Lee CT, Hilton S, Russo P. Renal mass within a horseshoe kidney: preoperative evaluation with three-dimensional helical computed tomography. *Urology*. 2001;57:168.

9. Saxton HM. Opacification of collecting ducts at urography [Editorial]. *Radiology*. 1989;170:16–17.

10. Ginalski J, Spiegel T, Jaaeger P. Use of low-osmolality contrast medium does not increase prevalence of medullary sponge kidney. *Radiology*. 1992;182:311–314.

11. Binder R, Korobkin M, Clark RE, et al. Aberrant papillae and other filling defects of the renal pelvis. *Am J Roentgenol*. 1972;114: 746–752.

12. Schwartz BB, Mindelzun RE. Ectopic (intrapelvic) renal papilla. *J Urol*. 1972;108:28–29.

13. Nino-Murcia M, Friedland GW, DeVries PA. Congenital anomalies of the papillae, calyces, renal pelvis, ureter, and ureteral orifice. In: Pollack HM, McClennan BL, eds. *Clinical urology*. 2nd ed. Philadelphia: Saunders; 2000:764–825.

14. Zagoria RJ. The renal sinus, pelvocalyceal system, and ureter. In: Zagoria RJ, ed. *The requisites: genitourinary radiology*. 2nd ed. Philadelphia: Mosby; 2004:158–200.

15. Talner LB, O'Reilly PH, Wasserman NF. Specific causes of obstruction. In: Pollack HM, McClennan BL, eds. *Clinical urology*. 2nd ed. Philadelphia: Saunders; 2000:2000–2007.

16. Herman TE, McAlister WH. Radiographic manifestations of congenital anomalies of the lower urinary tract. *Radiol Clin North Am*. 1991;29:365–382.

CHAPTER FIVE
UROLITHIASIS

SATOMI KAWAMOTO, MD

ELLIOT K. FISHMAN, MD

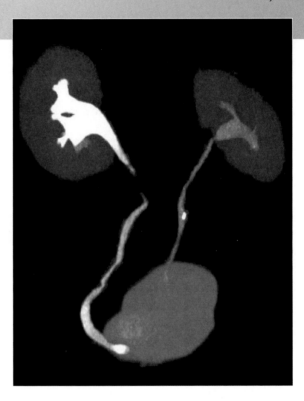

History: 76-year-old male with gross hematuria status post extracorporeal shock wave lithotripsy for urolithiasis.

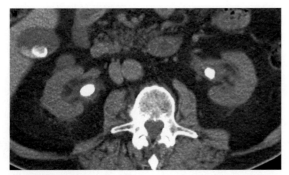

Figure 5.1   A

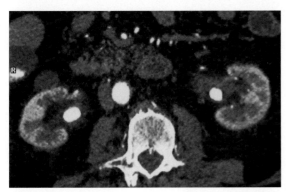

Figure 5.1   B

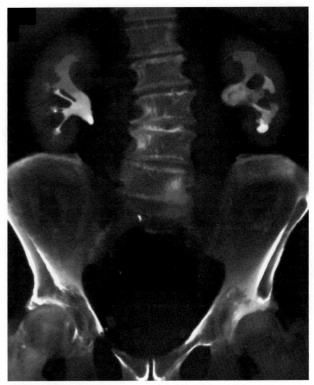

Figure 5.1   C

Findings: Unenhanced axial image (A) shows large calculi in the renal pelves. Gallstones are also present. Arterial phase axial image (B) again shows calculi in the renal pelves bilaterally. There is mild stranding of the fat surrounding the renal pelves. There is a cyst projecting off the anterior aspect of the right kidney. Excretory phase volume-rendered image (C) shows mild caliectasis bilaterally, left greater than right. The calculi are not visible because their attenuation values are similar to the attenuation of contrast material.

Diagnosis: Bilateral renal pelvis calculi with minimal hydronephrosis

Discussion: Urolithiasis is a common problem; the lifetime risk for stone disease in the urinary tract approaches 20% for males and 5% to 10% for females. The application of spiral (helical) CT for the diagnosis and management of urolithiasis has altered the practice of uroradiology dramatically. Prior to CT, the diagnosis of urolithiasis relied on plain radiography, intravenous urography, and ultrasound.

Almost three-fourths of urinary stones are composed of calcium oxalate, calcium phosphate, or both. Approximately 10% of stones contain no calcium; most of these calculi are composed primarily of uric acid or cystine. Pure uric acid stones are not visible with plain film radiography. However, almost all urinary calculi, including uric acid stones, are visible with unenhanced CT. There are a few exceptions; matrix stones and indinavir-induced stones are not of high attenuation on CT. Matrix stones are often seen as a nonenhancing soft tissue mass within the pelvicaliceal system. Indinavir is a protease inhibitor used in the treatment of HIV infection. Approximately 19% of the drug is excreted in the urine, and poorly soluble indinavir crystals act as nidi for stone formation. These stones are also of soft tissue attenuation.

History: 85-year-old male with recurrent gross hematuria.

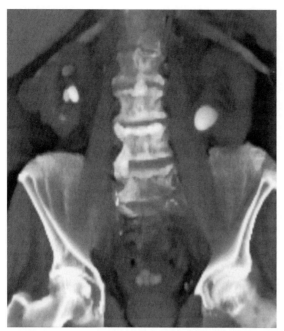

Figure 5.2   A

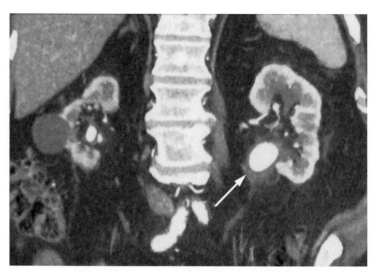

Figure 5.2   B

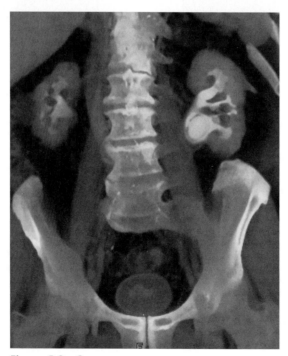

Figure 5.2   C

Findings: Unenhanced volume-rendered image from a CT urogram (A) shows a large calculus in the left renal pelvis. There are smaller calculi in the right renal pelvis, the upper and lower pole calices of the right kidney, and multiple calculi in the bladder. Arterial phase coronal image (B) again shows the large calculus in the dilated left renal pelvis and the smaller calculi in the right renal pelvis. The right kidney contains a cyst and is atrophic compared to the left kidney. There is thickening of both renal pelvic walls, more so on the left (arrow). Excretory phase volume-rendered image (C) shows mild caliectasis bilaterally. The large left renal pelvic calculus is again visualized because the dilated left renal pelvis is incompletely filled with excreted contrast at the time of the scan, but the right renal calculi are obscured by contrast material in the right renal collecting system. The multiple bladder calculi are also identified.

Diagnosis: Bilateral renal pelvis calculi and bladder calculi with associated pyelitis

Discussion: Chronically indwelling calculi may invoke an inflammatory reaction in the adjacent urothelium, with or without infection, and result in thickening of the urothelium and nearby fat stranding. The findings are indicative of pyelitis (see Case 8-6).

The bladder stones were not visible with plain radiographs and, therefore, were diagnosed as pure uric acid stones. The kidney stones were faintly seen by plain film and thought to be composed of both uric acid and a small amount of calcium. Cystoscopy confirmed the presence of multiple uric acid bladder stones. The patient underwent urinary alkalinization therapy, which significantly decreased stone burden, followed by extracorporeal shock wave lithotripsy. The left renal calculi were eventually found to be composed of 99% uric acid and 1% calcium oxalate monohydrate.

Pure uric acid stones are radiolucent on plain films but, as previously mentioned, easily visible on unenhanced CT images. In comparison, large uric acid stones may incorporate calcium and become radiopaque or serve as a nidus for calcium oxalate stones. Low urinary pH is a significant factor in the formation of uric acid calculi. Uric acid stones form in acidic urine; however, when the urine pH is increased to 6.5 or higher, uric acid has significantly increased solubility. This explains why urinary alkalinization is utilized to treat patients who develop uric acid stones.

History: 72-year-old male with a history of bladder and kidney stones.

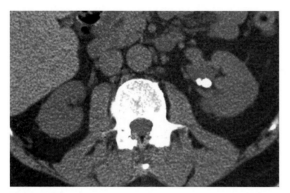

Figure 5.3   A

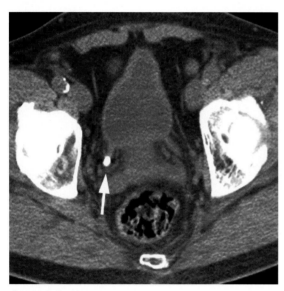

Figure 5.3   B

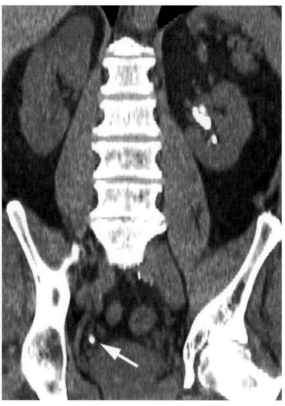

Figure 5.3   C

Findings: Unenhanced axial image (A) shows two contiguous calculi in the left renal pelvis. Unenhanced axial image through the pelvis (B) shows a calculus (arrow) in the distal right ureter. Unenhanced coronal reformatted image (C) shows multiple calculi in the renal pelvis and lower pole calyx of the left kidney and the small calculus (arrow) in the distal right ureter. There is no evidence of hydronephrosis or hydroureter.

Diagnosis: Left renal calculi and right distal ureteral calculus, without obstruction

Discussion: Virtually all ureteral calculi originate in the renal medulla or intrarenal collecting system. Stones in the ureter may be nonobstructing, but more commonly they obstruct and result in proximal hydronephrosis.

Calcifications adjacent to the ureter, such as arterial calcifications or phleboliths, may be difficult to differentiate from ureteral calculi, particularly when ureteral calculi are distal and nonobstructing and when the nondilated ureter cannot be identified in the lower abdomen and pelvis. The "soft tissue rim sign" caused by a thickened edematous ureteral wall around a ureteral stone can be seen in 50% to 77% of ureteral calculi but is not present around phleboliths. As a result, identification of the soft tissue rim sign allows for ureteral calculi to be distinguished definitively from phleboliths. Because some ureteral calculi do not cause ureteral wall edema, the absence of the soft tissue rim sign cannot be used to exclude a ureteral stone. A pelvic density without a rim could represent either a phlebolith or a ureteral calculus. Furthermore, the intraureteral nature of most calculi that demonstrate the soft tissue rim sign is usually otherwise obvious in most patients due to the presence of other signs of urinary tract obstruction, including pelvocaliectasis, ureterectasis, and perinephric and periureteric stranding and fluid.

In this patient, the right ureter was slightly dilated and the intraureteral location of the calculus could be identified without the aid of the soft tissue rim sign. Subsequently, the right ureteral calculus was removed ureteroscopically with laser lithotripsy.

CASE 5-4

History: 87-year-old male with right hip pain and hematuria. Urinalysis revealed a urinary tract infection.

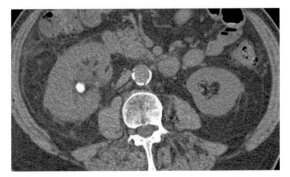

Figure 5.4   A

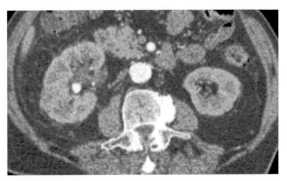

Figure 5.4   B

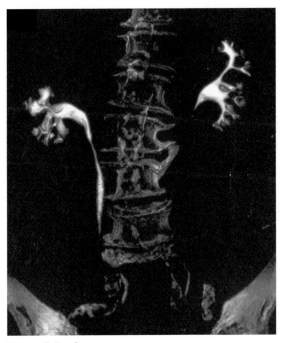

Figure 5.4   C

Findings: Unenhanced axial image from a CT urogram (A) shows a calculus in the right renal pelvis. The right kidney is enlarged, and there is more perinephric stranding on the right than on the left. Arterial phase axial image (B) shows the calculus in the right renal pelvis. Enlargement of the right kidney and perinephric stranding are again seen. Excretory phase volume-rendered image (C) shows minimal caliectasis on the right. The calculus in the right renal pelvis is obscured by excreted contrast material.

Diagnosis: Right renal pelvic calculus and probable acute pyelonephritis

Discussion: Most complications of urolithiasis are a result of obstruction or infection. Renal enlargement and perinephric stranding are signs of obstruction, infection, or both.

Pyelonephritis and its sequelae, such as intrarenal abscess, are common in patients with obstructing calculi, and when the clinical history and CT findings are appropriate, the diagnosis of pyelonephritis can be suggested. Acute pyelonephritis is characterized by fever, flank pain, bacteriuria, and pyuria. CT may show global enlargement of the affected kidney and patchy or wedge-shaped areas of decreased contrast enhancement. These findings are best seen on nephrographic phase images.

CASE 5-5

History: 43-year-old male with severe left flank pain that improved suddenly.

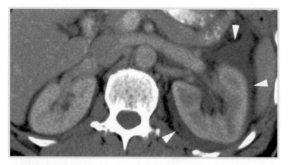

Figure 5.5   A

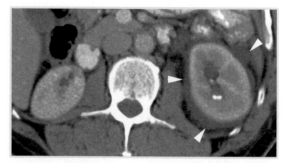

Figure 5.5   B

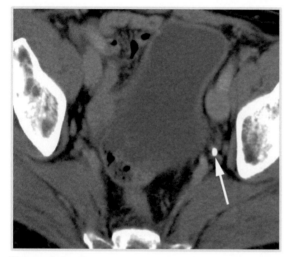

Figure 5.5   C

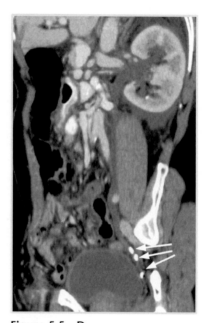

Figure 5.5   D

Findings: Nephrographic phase axial images (A, B) show mild hydronephrosis and delayed contrast enhancement of the left kidney. Small nonobstructing calculi are seen in the lower pole calyx of the left kidney on image (B). There is moderate fluid attenuation material around the left kidney (arrowheads). Nephrographic phase axial image of the pelvis (C) shows a calculus in the left distal ureter (arrow). Nephrographic phase curved planar reformatted image (D) shows that there are three calculi in the left distal ureter (arrows) with minimal left hydronephrosis and hydroureter. The fluid attenuation material around the left kidney is again seen.

Diagnosis: Nonobstructing calculi in the lower pole calyx of the left kidney and obstructing left distal ureteral calculi with forniceal rupture

Discussion: Obstructing ureteral calculi are most commonly located at or near the ureterovesical junction. Other common locations include the ureteropelvic junction and where the ureter crosses the iliac vessels. Acute ureteral obstruction causes severe flank pain also known as renal or ureteral colic. Renal colic is due to sudden distention of the proximal collecting system and edema of the kidney, exacerbated by ureteral hyperperistalsis. The combination of severe flank pain accompanied by hematuria is seen in approximately 50% of patients with ureterolithiasis.

For evaluation of renal colic, unenhanced CT or the first scan of a three-phase CT urogram is the study of choice. Contrast-enhanced CT scans are rarely needed. In one study, sensitivity and specificity of unenhanced CT for diagnosis of ureteral calculus in the emergency setting were 97% and 96%, respectively. In acute obstruction caused by a ureteral calculus, CT usually shows the obstructing calculus as well as secondary signs of obstruction, including hydroureter, hydronephrosis, perinephric stranding, and renal enlargement.

Occasionally, the obstructed collecting system can decompress spontaneously by leakage of urine from the renal collecting system, typically from one or more caliceal fornices. The fornix of the calyx is the weakest point of the renal collecting system. Rupture of the caliceal fornix may occur either as a result of a rapid increase in pressure in the renal collecting system due to acute urinary obstruction or during injection of contrast material directly into the renal collecting system during antegrade or retrograde pyelography. In most cases, the resulting extravasated urine tracks into the renal sinus. On delayed phase images of CT urography, the extravasated opacified contrast material may surround the renal pelvis and proximal ureter and extend further in the perinephric space (see Case 9-18). During antegrade and retrograde pyelography, contrast material extravasation occurs as a result of increased pressure and subsequent "backflow" phenomena. In this setting, forniceal rupture results in pyelosinus backflow or pyelosinus extravasation.

As a result of forniceal rupture, the obstructed collecting system becomes decompressed suddenly and, therefore, the patient's symptoms may improve abruptly. The treating physician may then assume falsely that the obstructing stone has passed. Forniceal rupture due to acute urinary obstruction usually has no clinical significance if the urine is not infected. The fluid will resolve over time, particularly if the urinary tract obstruction is relieved. (Case courtesy of Stuart G. Silverman, MD, Brigham and Women's Hospital, Boston, MA.)

CASE 5-6

History: 66-year-old male with hematuria.

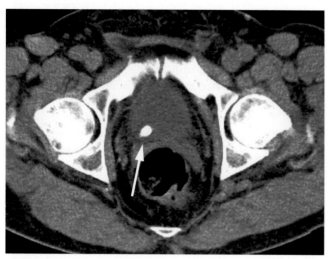

Figure 5.6   A

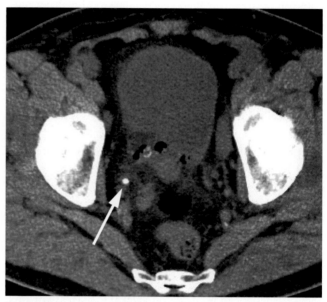

Figure 5.6   B

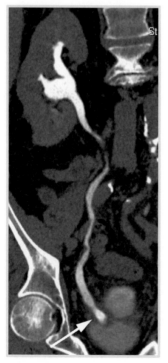

Figure 5.6   C

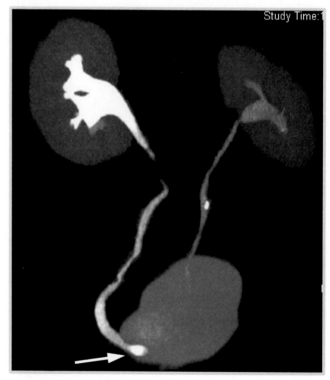

Figure 5.6   D

Findings: Unenhanced axial image of the pelvis from a CT urogram (A) shows a 1-cm calculus at the right ureterovesical junction (arrow). Unenhanced axial image of the pelvis more superiorly (B) shows an additional 4-mm calculus in the right distal ureter, 1.5 cm above the ureterovesical junction (arrow). Excretory phase coronal (C) and MIP (D) images show mild right-sided hydronephrosis and hydroureter. The calculus at the right ureterovesical junction is well-visualized (arrow); however, the smaller calculus in the right distal ureter located more superiorly is obscured by excreted contrast material.

Diagnosis: Obstructing calculi at the distal ureter and right ureterovesical junction

Discussion: Projectional techniques, including three-dimensional imaging, multiplanar reformation, and curved planar reformation, are helpful for evaluation of the size and extent of the stones. Measurement of maximal stone diameter can be used to predict the likelihood of stone passage. Larger stones, particularly those measuring >5 mm in diameter, are less likely to pass than stones <5 mm. Size measurements can be made on axial CT images; however, the longest dimension of a calculus is usually in the z-axis, and z-axis measurements are most easily made on reformatted coronal or sagittal images.

When attenuation of the calculi and excreted contrast material within the renal collecting system and ureter are different, calculi are visualized on excretory phase images of a CT urogram. Maximum intensity images are particularly useful in depicting calculi during the excretory phase. However, regardless of the reconstruction technique used, excreted contrast material can obscure stones when attenuation of the calculi and the contrast material are similar.

When a calculus is seen in or immediately adjacent to the ureterovesical junction, particularly on unenhanced CT images, it can be difficult to differentiate stones impacted at the ureterovesical junction from stones that have already passed into the bladder. Prone images can be used to make this distinction. Stones that have passed into the bladder will fall dependently to the anterior aspect of the bladder when the patient is placed in the prone position, whereas stones impacted at the ureterovesical junction will remain unchanged. (Case courtesy of Stuart G. Silverman, MD, Brigham and Women's Hospital, Boston, MA.)

History: 56-year-old male with a 3-day history of right-sided abdominal and flank pain, worsening nausea and vomiting, and dehydration.

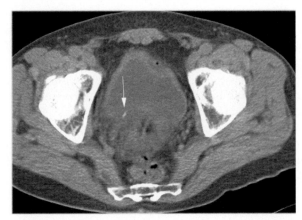

Figure 5.7 A

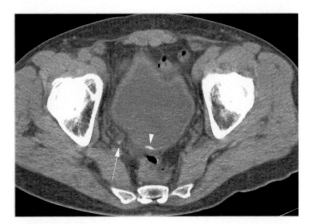

Figure 5.7 B

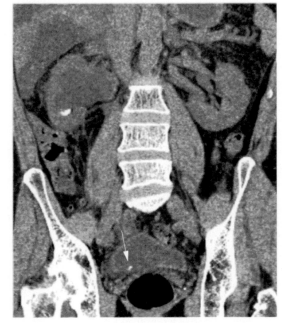

Figure 5.7 C

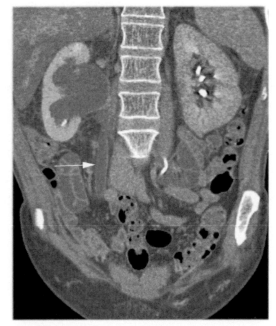

Figure 5.7 D

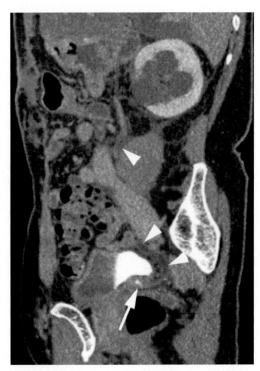

Figure 5.7 E

Findings: Unenhanced axial image through the lower pelvis (A) shows a small calculus at the right ureterovesical junction (arrow). Unenhanced axial image of the pelvis (B) slightly higher than (A) shows an additional tiny calculus in the distal right ureter (arrow). A small calculus (arrowhead) is also seen in the dependent portion of the bladder. Unenhanced coronal image (C) shows moderate right hydronephrosis and another small calculus in a dilated right renal collecting system. The small right ureterovesical junction calculus seen in (A) is again visualized (arrow). Excretory phase coronal image (D) shows moderate right hydronephrosis and hydroureter (arrow) and delayed excretion of contrast material from the right kidney. Excretory phase oblique lateral posterior image through the right kidney (E) shows that the dilated right ureter (arrowheads) extends to the calculus (arrow) at the ureterovesical junction.

Diagnosis: Calculi in the right renal collecting system, right distal ureter, and bladder, with ureteral obstruction due to the calculus at the ureterovesical junction

Discussion: Most small ureteral calculi pass spontaneously without obstruction. Obstructing distal ureteral calculi that are <5 mm generally pass spontaneously; these calculi can usually be managed effectively without intervention. Because the ureteral calculi were small in this patient, he was initially managed with intravenous fluids and observation alone. However, the patient's discomfort continued. Therefore, cystoscopy and ureteroscopy was performed. The distal ureter contained no calculi; presumably, the obstructing calculi had passed spontaneously. Numerous bladder calculi were found.

CASE 5-8

History: 71-year-old male with hematuria.

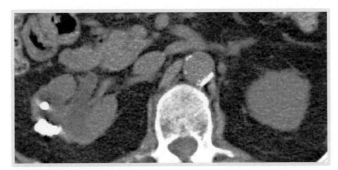

Figure 5.8   A

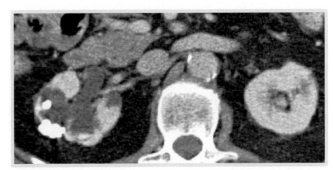

Figure 5.8   B

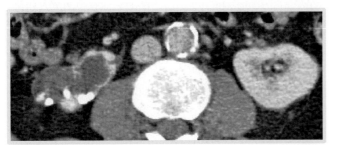

Figure 5.8   C

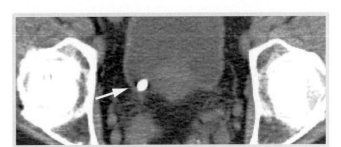

Figure 5.8   D

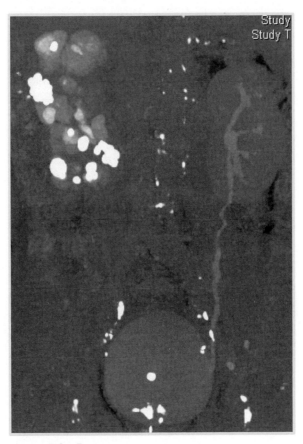

Figure 5.8   E

Findings: Unenhanced (A) and nephrographic phase (B) axial images from a CT urogram show moderate to severe right hydronephrosis with multiple stones in dilated calices. The right renal parenchyma is atrophic, suggesting that the hydronephrosis and obstruction has probably been long-standing. Nephrographic phase axial image obtained more inferiorly (C) again shows hydronephrosis and marked parenchymal atrophy of the right kidney. The left kidney is normal. The right ureter is not dilated. An unenhanced image of the pelvis (D) shows additional 7-mm calculus in the region of the right ureterovesical junction (arrow). Excretory phase maximum intensity projection (MIP) image (E) shows multiple dilated right renal calices containing multiple stones.

Diagnosis: Long-standing right hydronephrosis probably due to chronic ureteropelvic junction obstruction, with multiple calculi within the dilated calices and a large calculus at the right ureterovesical junction

Discussion: In the setting of chronic urinary obstruction, atrophy of renal parenchyma may occur due to increased hydrostatic pressure on renal tissue and ischemia from compression of intrarenal arteries and veins. These changes typically involve the entire affected kidney.

Because the right ureter is not dilated, the long-standing hydronephrosis is probably due to obstruction at the level of the ureteropelvic junction. The presence of ureteropelvic junction obstruction and simultaneous stone disease is common, with prior studies reporting a 20% incidence of stones in these patients. Stones that develop as a result of chronic obstruction, as in this case, are considered to be secondary urolithiasis. Calculi may be located in a calyx, free floating in the renal pelvis, or impacted at the uretero-pelvic junction. When the stones become impacted, they may exacerbate the already present obstruction. (Case courtesy of Stuart G. Silverman, MD, Brigham and Women's Hospital, Boston, MA.)

History: 71-year-old male presented with hematuria and a history of a left-sided pelvic kidney, status post previous open left renal surgery for recurrent left renal pelvic stones. The patient is also status post abdominal aortic aneurysm repair with left renal artery graft.

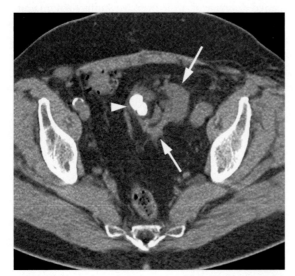

Figure 5.9 A

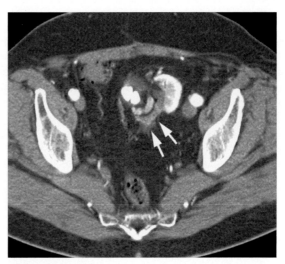

Figure 5.9 B

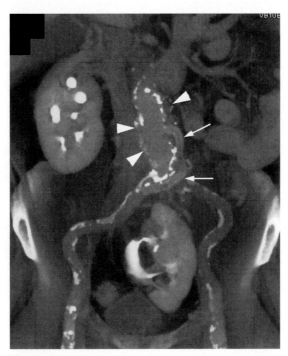

Figure 5.9 C

Findings: Unenhanced axial image of the pelvis from a CT urogram (A) shows an ectopically located left-sided pelvic kidney (arrows) containing two large calculi (arrowhead) in the renal pelvis. The left kidney is atrophic and there is minimal perinephric stranding. Arterial phase axial image (B) shows the pelvic kidney with a large area of parenchymal scarring and hypoperfusion posteriorly (arrows). Excretory phase volume-rendered image (C) shows that there is no hydronephrosis or hydroureter. The calculi are obscured by the excreted contrast material. The right kidney is located in a normal position but is malrotated. The left renal artery graft (arrows) is identified, as are postsurgical changes from the aortic aneurysm repair (arrowheads). Extensive atherosclerotic calcification is seen in the lower abdominal aorta and iliac vessels.

Diagnosis: Pelvic left kidney with multiple nonobstructing calculi in the left renal pelvis

Discussion: Abnormalities of ascent, formation, or fusion of the kidneys during embryologic development can result in anomalous kidney position. Horseshoe kidney and pelvic kidney are the most frequently encountered congenital abnormalities of ascent.

Relative to the rest of the population, stones are more common in patients with horseshoe and pelvic kidneys. It has been postulated that as a result of an anteriorly located renal pelvis and renal malrotation in patients with these anomalies, there is impaired drainage of urine from the kidney. Anomalous vasculature may also inhibit drainage by partially compressing the ureter at the ureteropelvic junction. Altered anatomy may present a significant challenge to the urologist caring for patients with symptomatic urolithiasis. Stone extraction procedures may be considerably more complex. CT urography may help in planning surgical and/or interventional treatment.

CASE 5-10

History: 30-year-old female with a history of right pelvic kidney and intermittent lower back pain that has become worse during the past few months.

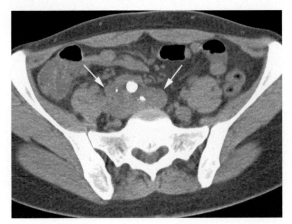

Figure 5.10   A

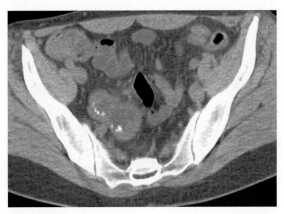

Figure 5.10   B

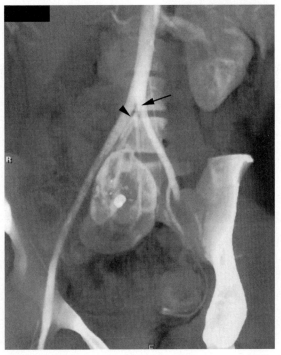

Figure 5.10   C

Findings: Unenhanced axial image of the pelvis (A) shows a right-sided pelvic kidney (arrows) with a large calculus in the renal pelvis and smaller caliceal calculi. Unenhanced axial image obtained slightly more inferiorly (B) shows multiple small calculi in the dependent portions of dilated calices in the lower pole of the pelvic kidney. Arterial phase volume-rendered image (C) shows the large calculus in the right renal pelvis as well as numerous other calculi scattered throughout the kidney. The right renal artery (arrow) originates from the distal abdominal aorta just proximal to its bifurcation and has an early bifurcation (arrowhead) as well. The left kidney has a normal position.

Diagnosis: Pelvic right kidney with multiple calculi, including a large obstructing renal pelvic calculus

Discussion: This case illustrates another patient with a pelvic kidney who developed nephrolithiasis, as previously mentioned, a known complication of renal position anomalies (see Case 5-9). In this patient, the stones were removed and a pyeloplasty was performed for a concomitant ureteropelvic junction obstruction.

History: 49-year-old female with a history of nephrolithiasis and a pelvic kidney.

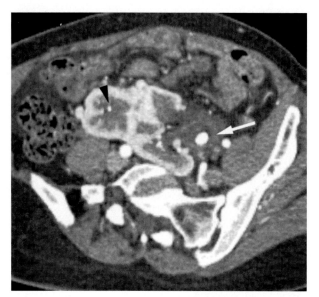

Figure 5.11   A

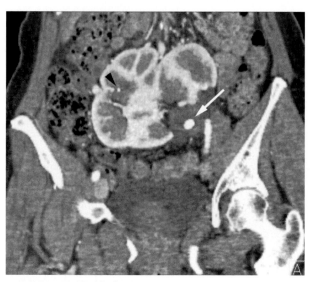

Figure 5.11   B

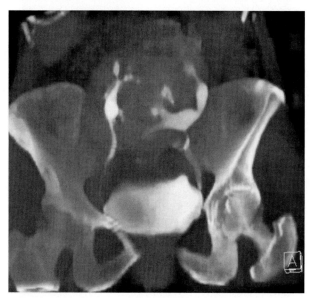

Figure 5.11   C

Findings: Arterial phase oblique axial (A) and coronal (B) images from a CT urogram show a fused pelvic kidney with an appearance compatible with lump or cake kidney. There is a large calculus in the pelvis of the left renal moiety (arrow) and a small caliceal calculus in the right renal moiety (arrowhead). Thickening of the pelvis of the left renal moiety and stranding are present also. An excretory phase volume-rendered image (C) shows a fused single pelvic kidney with separate renal collecting systems and ureters. The calculi are obscured by excreted contrast material.

Diagnosis: Pelvic lump or cake kidney containing multiple calculi

Discussion: There are several types of fusion anomalies of the kidneys. When the kidneys are joined at the medial borders of each upper and lower pole to produce a doughnut- or ring-shaped mass, they are classified as doughnut kidney. When there is more extensive fusion along the entire medial aspect of each kidney, they produce a disc or shield kidney. In a disc or shield kidney, the lateral aspect of each kidney retains its normal contour, and the reniform shape is preserved more than in the lump or cake kidney. The lump or cake kidney is a relatively rare fusion anomaly. Extensive joining has taken place over a wide margin of the maturing renal anlage, and the total kidney mass is irregular and lobulated. In many instances, the kidney remains within the pelvis. Both renal pelves are anterior in location, and they drain separate areas of parenchyma.

Most patients with fusion anomalies are asymptomatic, but hydronephrosis and renal calculi can occur. In this patient, renal calculi are noted in both moieties. Thickening and stranding of the pelvis of the left renal moiety are due to pyelitis caused by the large left renal pelvic calculus.

History: 61-year-old male with fever, status post radical cystectomy and ileal conduit for bladder cancer.

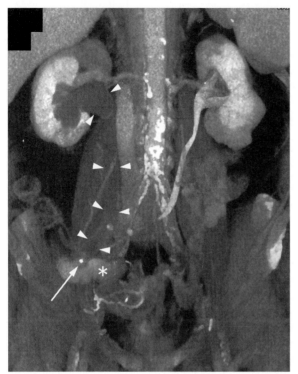

Figure 5.12   A

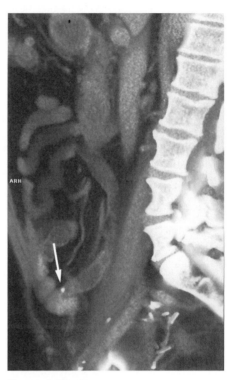

Figure 5.12   B

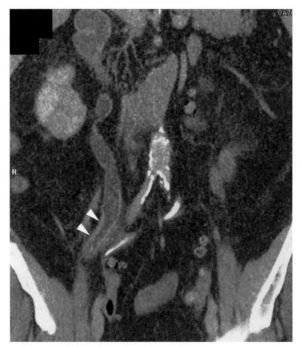

Figure 5.12   C

Findings: Excretory phase volume-rendered image from a CT urogram (A) shows moderate right hydronephrosis and hydroureter (arrowheads) that extends to an ileal conduit (asterisk) in the right lower quadrant. There is delayed excretion of contrast material into the right renal collecting system and ureter. A small calculus (arrow) is seen in the distal right ureter at the level of the right ureteroileal anastomosis. Excretory phase oblique sagittal volume-rendered image (B) again shows the small calculus (arrow) in the distal right ureter at the level of the right ureteroileal anastomosis. Excretory phase coronal image (C) shows that the distal right ureter is thickened and dilated (arrowheads).

Diagnosis: Obstructing distal right ureteral calculus status post cystectomy and ileal loop urinary diversion

Discussion: Patients who undergo urinary tract diversion procedures have an increased risk of developing urolithiasis. In fact, urolithiasis is seen in 10% to 12% of patients with ileal conduits. In this patient, ureteroscopy was subsequently performed, and a small stone was removed from the distal right ureter. A right ureteral stricture was also identified at the ileal anastomosis. The patient then underwent excision of the stricture and revision of the ureteroenteric anastomosis. At pathology, there was mild chronic inflammation and serosal fibrosis at the stricture site, without evidence of malignancy.

History: 54-year-old male status post ileocolonic resection for Crohn disease has a history of multiple vascular thromboses. CT was performed to determine whether a vascular thrombosis was present; there were no urinary complaints.

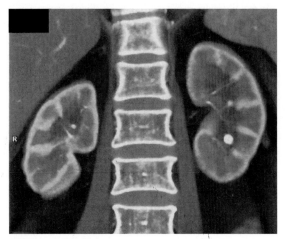

Figure 5.13   A

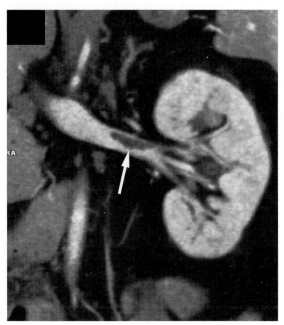

Figure 5.13   C

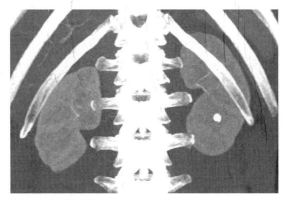

Figure 5.13   B

Findings: Corticomedullary phase volume-rendered image (A) and nephrographic phase maximum intensity projection image (B) show an 8-mm nonobstructing calculus in the lower pole of the left kidney. Nephrographic phase volume-rendered image (C) shows a nonocclusive thrombus in the left renal vein (arrow).

Diagnosis: Left-sided nephrolithiasis and renal vein thrombosis in a patient with Crohn disease

Discussion: Crohn disease is associated with increased renal stone formation; stones are found in 3.2% to 8.6% of patients. Most contain calcium; however, 29% are uric acid calculi. There are two mechanisms for renal stone formation in patients with Crohn disease. Chronic volume contraction in these patients may result from losses of both water and salt in the stool. This leads to decreased urine volumes and the precipitation of calcium oxalate stones. The urine also tends to be acidic due to excessive bicarbonate losses in the stool. Acidic urine leads to uric acid stone formation. Patients with Crohn disease may also develop secondary oxalosis. This occurs in patients with diseased distal small bowel, who have relatively normal colonic mucosa. In this setting, excess amounts of oxalate are reabsorbed. Patients with secondary oxalosis also may develop nephrocalcinosis (which is often of the "cortical" type).

Urinary tract stones are also more common in patients with chronic diarrhea of other etiologies and in patients who have undergone gastrointestinal surgery, especially in the presence of an ileostomy.

CASE 5-14

History: 57-year-old female with history of nephrolithiasis.

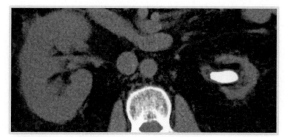

Figure 5.14 A

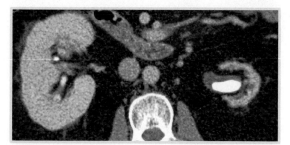

Figure 5.14 B

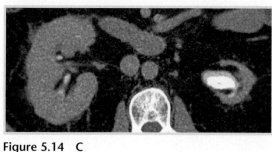

Figure 5.14 C

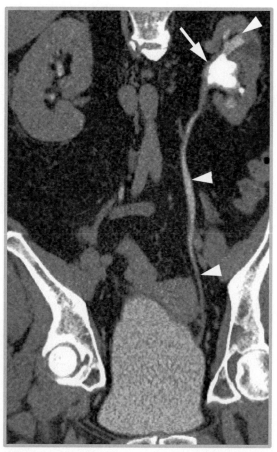

Figure 5.14 D

Findings: Unenhanced (A), nephrographic (B), and excretory phase (C) axial images from a CT urogram show a large calculus in the left renal pelvis. The left kidney is markedly atrophic. The right kidney is enlarged due to compensatory hypertrophy. Excretory phase curved planar reformatted image (D) again shows the large calculus (arrow) in the left renal pelvis. The calculus has a higher attenuation than excreted contrast material in the renal collecting system and ureter (arrowheads) and is therefore well-visualized on the excretory phase image.

Diagnosis: Large calculus in the left renal pelvis with marked atrophy of the left kidney and compensatory hypertrophy of the right kidney

Discussion: With long-term uninfected obstruction, atrophy of the kidney may result with subsequent inability to resume normal function once the obstruction is relieved. Hypertrophy of the contralateral kidney may compensate for the absence or the diminished function of a kidney. In this patient, the large calculus in the left renal pelvis is visualized well on both axial and reformatted excretory phase images because the attenuation of the calculus is higher than the attenuation of excreted contrast material within the collecting system and ureter (also discussed in Case 5-6). In this case, the stone is easier to visualize because the attenuation of the opacified urine was lowered by intravenous furosemide used adjunctively to improve opacification and distension of the collecting systems and ureters during CT urography. (Case courtesy of Stuart G. Silverman, MD, Brigham and Women's Hospital, Boston, MA.)

History: 40-year-old female with a 3-year history of kidney stones, now with left-sided flank pain.

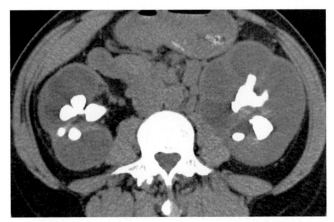

Figure 5.15 A

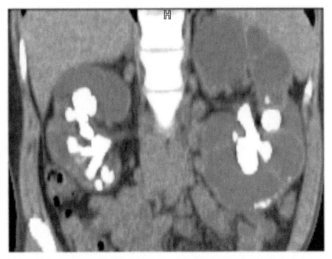

Figure 5.15 B

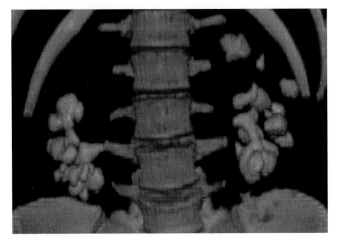

Figure 5.15 C

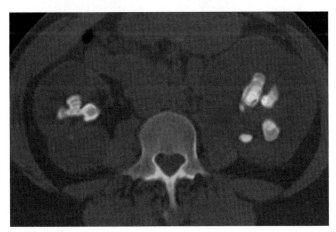

Figure 5.15 D

Findings: Unenhanced axial (A) and coronal (B) images of the kidneys show large bilateral obstructing staghorn calculi. There is marked thinning of the renal parenchyma and severe hydronephrosis bilaterally. Unenhanced anterior coronal image (B) shows marked thinning of the renal parenchyma and hypoattenuating areas between the parenchyma and staghorn calculi. Unenhanced volume-rendered image with thresholds such that only high attenuation staghorn calculi (and bones) can be visualized (C). Unenhanced axial image through the kidney with a wide window setting (D) shows that these calculi demonstrate a laminated appearance due to alternating bands of different attenuation.

Diagnosis: Bilateral staghorn calculi and xanthogranulomatous pyelonephritis

Discussion: Staghorn calculi are, by definition, confined to and fill the intrarenal collecting system. Approximately 70% of staghorn calculi are composed of struvite. The remaining staghorn calculi are composed of cystine or uric acid. Struvite stones are frequently associated with infected urine and are usually mixed with calcium phosphate (apatite) to form the so-called triple phosphate stone (magnesium–ammonium–calcium phosphate). *Proteus, Pseudomonas, Klebsiella,* and *Staphylococcus* bacterial species are capable of producing urease, an enzyme that splits urea and forms ammonia. Because ammonia is a weak base, these organisms lead to alkalinization of urine, which promotes the precipitation of magnesium ammonium phosphate crystals. Struvite stones have a laminated appearance because calcium phosphate often precipitates between the magnesium ammonium phosphate components in layers.

Xanthogranulomatous pyelonephritis is a rare chronic renal infection that typically results from long-standing obstruction (see Cases 6-14 and 8-19). At pathology, the renal parenchyma is replaced by yellow-colored masses, which are composed of foamy lipid-laden macrophages, other inflammatory cells, and fibrosis. There are two forms of the disease. The diffuse form often results in complete loss of function of the affected kidney. A less common focal form presents as an inflammatory mass. In adults, more than 70% of patients with the diffuse form of xanthogranulomatous pyelonephritis present with an obstructing staghorn or ureteral calculus, generally composed of struvite, and marked hydronephrosis, as in this case. Occasionally, the inflammatory process may extend into the psoas muscle and perirenal and pararenal spaces. Perinephric fluid collections may be successfully treated with percutaneous catheter drainage; however, the kidney usually remains a nidus for infection and total nephrectomy is often eventually required.

In this case, bilateral nephrostomies were placed; the right one drained purulent material. Renal imaging using Tc-99m dimercaptosuccinic acid (DMSA) revealed no function on the right and poor function on the left. Subsequent right nephrectomy revealed xanthogranulomatous pyelonephritis.

History: 40-year-old female with a history of distal renal tubular acidosis, recurrent urinary tract infections, and right-sided flank pain.

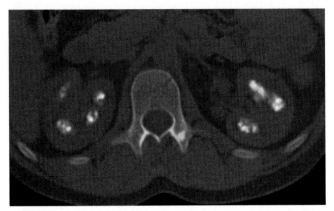

Figure 5.16   A

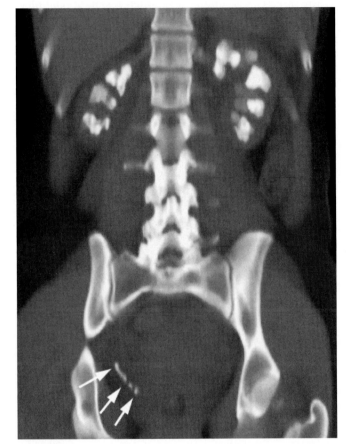

Figure 5.16   B

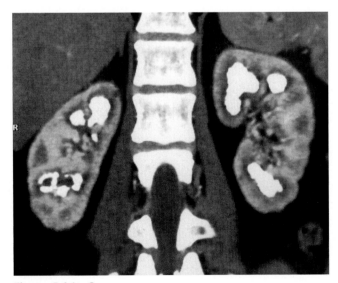

Figure 5.16   C

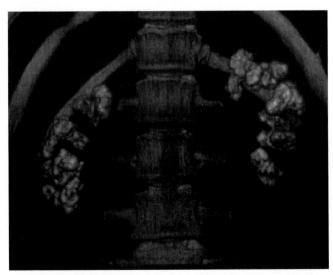

Figure 5.16   D

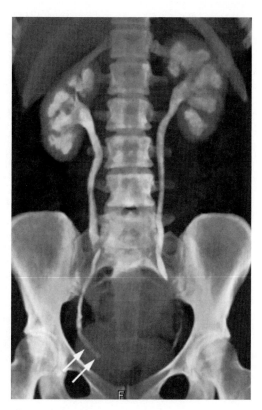

Figure 5.16   E

Findings: Unenhanced axial image of the kidneys obtained at CT urography with a wide window setting (A) shows extensive calcifications in the medulla of both kidneys and parenchymal thinning. Unenhanced volume-rendered image (B) also shows extensive calcifications in the medulla of both kidneys as well as multiple calculi in the distal right ureter (arrows). Arterial phase coronal reformatted (C) and volume-rendered (D) images also show medullary calcifications. The excretory phase volume-rendered image (E) shows the calcifications, although they are difficult to differentiate from the intrarenal collecting systems. The right ureter is also minimally dilated due to the right distal ureteral calculi (arrows).

Diagnosis: Medullary nephrocalcinosis secondary to distal renal tubular acidosis and obstructing distal right ureteral calculi

Discussion: There are two major types of involvement of the urinary tract by calculus disease: (i) nephrocalcinosis, which represents the formation of concretions within the renal parenchyma, and (ii) urolithiasis, which represents stones within the lumen of the urinary tract. These two categories overlap because small stones that form in the distal tubules may erode into the collecting system. In cases of medullary nephrocalcinosis, stippled calcifications are seen in the distal tubules in the region of the renal pyramids. These calcium concretions may be small and poorly defined or they may be large and coarse. The most common etiology of medullary nephrocalcinosis is hyperparathyroidism (approximately 40%). Approximately 20% is caused by renal tubular acidosis, 20% by renal tubular ectasia, and the remainder by a variety of causes, including other hypercalcemic states. In the distal (type I) form of renal tubular acidosis, the distal renal tubules cannot effectively secrete hydrogen ions to lower the urinary pH. As a result, the urinary pH is higher than normal and stones precipitate and form in the tubules. Renal tubular acidosis is capable of causing exuberant nephrocalcinosis. In fact, when extensive medullary nephrocalcinosis is seen, renal tubular acidosis is usually the underlying cause.

SUGGESTED READINGS

1. Amis ESJ, Newhouse JH. Urinary stone disease. In: Amis ESJ, Newhouse JH, eds. *Essentials of uroradiology*. Boston: Little, Brown; 1991:153–170.

2. Liu CC, Li CC, Shih MC, et al. Matrix stone. *J Comput Assist Tomogr*. 2003;27:810–813.

3. Schwartz BF, Schenkman N, Armenakas NA, et al. Imaging characteristics of indinavir calculi. *J Urol*. 1999;161:1085–1087.

4. Blake SP, McNicholas MM, Raptopoulos V. Nonopaque crystal deposition causing ureteric obstruction in patients with HIV undergoing indinavir therapy. *Am J Roentgenol*. 1998;171:717–720.

5. Bell TV, Fenlon HM, Davison BD, et al. Unenhanced helical CT criteria to differentiate distal ureteral calculi from pelvic phleboliths. *Radiology*. 1998;207:363–367.

6. Kawashima A, Sandler CM, Boridy IC, et al. Unenhanced helical CT of ureterolithiasis: value of the tissue rim sign. *Am J Roentgenol*. 1997;168:997–1000.

7. Heneghan JP, Dalrymple NC, Verga M, et al. Soft-tissue "rim" sign in the diagnosis of ureteral calculi with use of unenhanced helical CT. *Radiology*. 1997;202:709–711.

8. Davidson AJ. *Davidson's radiology of the kidney and genitourinary tract*. 3rd ed. Philadelphia: Saunders; 1999.

9. Smith RC, Verga M, McCarthy S, et al. Diagnosis of acute flank pain: value of unenhanced helical CT. *Am J Roentgenol*. 1996;166:97–101.

10. Smith RC, Verga M, Dalrymple N, et al. Acute ureteral obstruction: value of secondary signs of helical unenhanced CT. *Am J Roentgenol*. 1996;167:1109–1113.

11. Levine J, Neitlich J, Smith RC. The value of prone scanning to distinguish ureterovesical junction stones from ureteral stones that have passed into the bladder: leave no stone unturned. *Am J Roentgenol*. 1999;172:977–981.

12. Dalrymple NC, Verga M, Anderson KR, et al. The value of unenhanced helical computerized tomography in the management of acute flank pain. *J Urol*. 1998;159:735–740.

13. Coll DM, Varanelli MJ, Smith RC. Relationship of spontaneous passage of ureteral calculi to stone size and location as revealed by unenhanced helical CT. *Am J Roentgenol*. 2002;178:101–103.

14. Takahashi N, Kawashima A, Ernst RD, et al. Ureterolithiasis: can clinical outcome be predicted with unenhanced helical CT? *Radiology*. 1998;208:97–102.

15. Rutchik SD, Resnick MI. Ureteropelvic junction obstruction and renal calculi. Pathophysiology and implications for management. *Urol Clin North Am*. 1998;25:317–321.

16. Bauer SB. Anomalies of the upper urinary tract. In: Walsh PC, ed. *Campbell's urology*. Philadelphia: Saunders; 2002.

17. Weizer AZ, Springhart WP, Ekeruo WO, et al. Ureteroscopic management of renal calculi in anomalous kidneys. *Urology*. 2005;65: 265–269.

18. Beiko DT, Razvi H. Stones in urinary diversions: update on medical and surgical issues. *Curr Opin Urol*. 2002;12:297–303.

19. Worcester EM. Stones from bowel disease. *Endocrinol Metab Clin North Am*. 2002;31:979–999.

20. Dunnick NR, Sandler CM, Amis ESJ, et al. Nephrocalcinosis and nephrolithiasis. In: Mitchell CW, ed. *Textbook of uroradiology*. Baltimore: Williams & Wilkins; 1997:254–281.

CHAPTER SIX
RENAL INFECTIONS

Sᴀᴍᴇʜ K. Mᴏʀᴄᴏs, MD, FRCS, FRCR

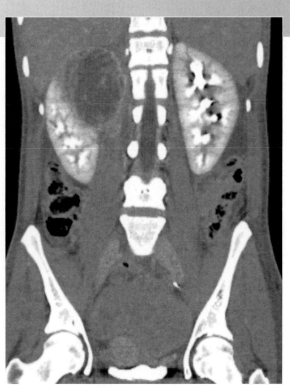

History: 26-year-old female with right flank pain, fever, nausea, and positive urine culture.

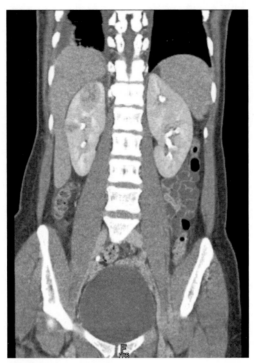

Figure 6.1

Findings: Coronal reformatted image from a CT urogram demonstrates a focal round low-attenuation area in the upper pole as well as a smaller area in the mid right kidney.

Diagnosis: Multifocal acute bacterial pyelonephritis

Discussion: Acute pyelonephritis is used to refer to an acute inflammatory infectious process affecting the renal parenchyma. Most affected patients are young or middle-aged women. Infection usually begins in the bladder and ascends to involve the ureters, intrarenal collecting systems, and then the kidneys. The most common offending organism is *Escherichia coli* (*E. coli*). On images obtained at CT urography, acute pyelonephritis may produce one or more focal, round areas of low attenuation, as in this case, or diffuse renal enlargement. Portions of the kidney may also show alternating linear areas of increased and decreased attenuation, creating a striated nephrogram. Treatment with antibiotics is usually effective; however, in some patients, antibiotic therapy may be needed for 6 to 8 weeks. (Case courtesy of Satomi Kawamoto, MD, Johns Hopkins Medical Institutions, Baltimore, MD.)

CASE 6-2

History: 33-year-old female with a history of tuberculosis presents with fever, left flank pain, and elevated white blood cell count.

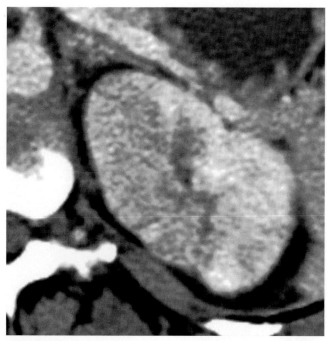

Figure 6.2

Findings: Axial image of the left kidney during the nephrographic phase obtained as part of a CT urogram shows an area of ill-defined, low density in the renal parenchyma.

Diagnosis: Acute pyelonephritis

Discussion: In patients with acute pyelonephritis, CT urography may demonstrate focal areas of low attenuation on nephrographic phase images. These areas of abnormally decreased enhancement may be patchy, round, or wedge shaped.

In comparison, delayed excretory phase images may reveal increased accumulation of contrast material in or adjacent to the abnormal previously hypodense parenchyma. CT urography in this case showed no signs of tuberculosis; the detected changes were compatible with the subsequently clinically established diagnosis of acute bacterial pyelonephritis. Tuberculosis typically produces more severe changes in the kidneys, including well-defined areas of low attenuation in the kidneys, renal parenchymal calcifications, and renal collecting system distortion and dilatation (see Cases 6-12 and 6-13). (Case courtesy of Stuart G. Silverman, MD, Brigham and Women's Hospital, Boston, MA.)

History: 30-year-old female with history of intravenous drug abuse presents with chills, right flank pain, and increased urinary frequency.

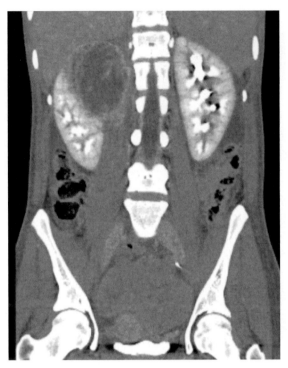

Figure 6.3   A

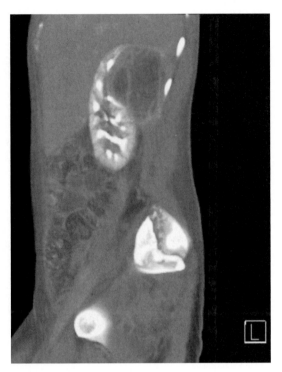

Figure 6.3   B

Findings: Coronal (A) and sagittal (B) enhanced images from a CT urogram show a 7-cm mass in the upper pole of the right kidney. The mass is predominantly hypodense with multiple enhancing septations, and it contains an irregularly thickened and enhancing wall.

Diagnosis: Renal abscess

Discussion: Although most acute renal infections resolve with antibiotic therapy, in some patients, particularly those who are immunosuppressed, renal abscesses may develop. Renal abscesses form in most patients as a result of inadequate treatment of an ascending infection, typically with *E. coli*. Intravenous drug abusers may develop renal abscesses as a result of hematogenous seeding. In these patients, *Staphylococcus, Streptococcus,* and *Enterobacter* species are more common than *E. coli*. On images obtained at CT urography, renal abscesses may have an appearance similar to that of a benign complicated renal cyst. In the appropriate setting, an abscess may be diagnosed when a cystic mass demonstrates a thickened, inflamed wall surrounding a hypodense fluid collection. Perinephric stranding, found commonly in the setting of inflammatory processes, is usually present and an important clue to the diagnosis. In this case, the abscess was due to *Staphylococcus aureus* and treated successfully with percutaneous CT-guided needle aspiration and catheter drainage. (Case courtesy of Satomi Kawamoto, MD, Johns Hopkins Medical Institutions, Baltimore, MD.)

History: 18-year-old male with right loin pain and recurrent fevers for 4 weeks despite antibiotics.

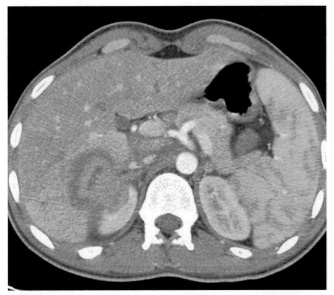

Figure 6.4   A

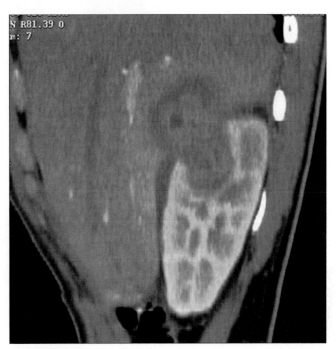

Figure 6.4   B

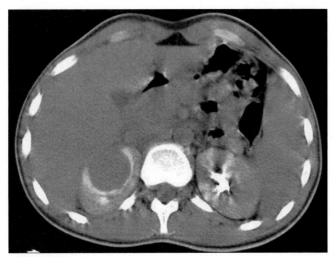

Figure 6.4   C

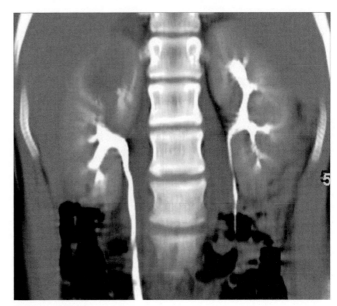

Figure 6.4   D

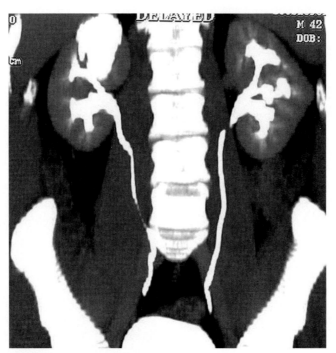

Figure 6.4   E

Findings: Axial (A) and sagittal (B) corticomedullary phase images from a CT urogram show a 4.5-cm mass involving the right kidney and a peripheral portion of adjacent liver. The mass has a thick enhancing wall and a nonenhancing, hypodense central portion. Early excretory phase images (C, D) demonstrate hyperenhancement of the adjacent renal parenchyma. Delayed (30-minute), thick coronal slab maximum intensity projection image (E) shows that the mass fills with contrast medium.

Diagnosis: Renal abscess

Discussion: If left untreated, renal abscesses may enlarge and spread locally. Renal abscesses may penetrate through the renal capsule into the perinephric space and result in perinephric abscess formation. Although uncommon, renal abscesses may also involve adjacent organs, as in this case, in which a portion of liver was involved. Finally, as this case demonstrates, a renal abscess may excavate into the collecting system. As a result, the abscess may be opacified with excreted contrast material on delayed excretory phase images. Urine culture is typically positive in patients with ascending urinary tract infections; however, it may be negative in patients who develop renal abscesses due to hematogenous seeding. The offending organism was not cultured in this case. (Case courtesy of Tarek El Diasty, MD, Mansoura University, Mansoura, Egypt.)

CASE 6-5

History: 32-year-old paraplegic male who developed a urinary tract infection and right flank pain despite prophylactic antibiotics.

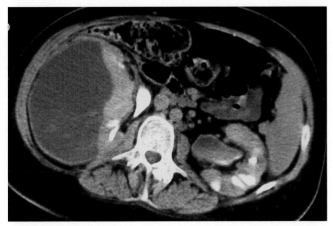

Figure 6.5   A

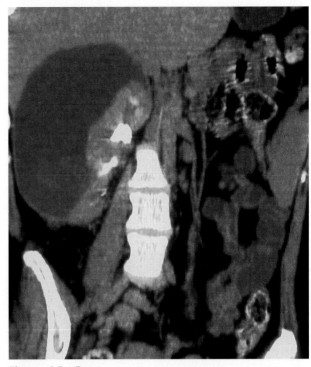

Figure 6.5   B

Findings: Axial (A) and coronal (B) excretory phase images from a CT urogram demonstrate a large, low-attenuation collection along the lateral aspect of the right kidney; the renal parenchyma is severely compressed. There is bilateral moderate caliectasis and multifocal renal parenchymal loss on the left, likely due to chronic pyelonephritis or reflux nephropathy.

Diagnosis: Subcapsular renal abscess

Discussion: Infected subcapsular fluid collections are an uncommon sequela of renal infection. They are best treated with percutaneous catheter drainage. CT urography can be used to demonstrate the subcapsular location of the fluid, determine its extent, and help plan the percutaneous drainage procedure. In this case, percutaneous catheter drainage yielded purulent material, although no organisms were identified (possibly because the patient was already being treated with antibiotics). The patient recovered following percutaneous drainage and continued treatment with broad-spectrum antibiotics.

CASE 6-6

History: 42-year-old female with pyuria, fever, and flank pain.

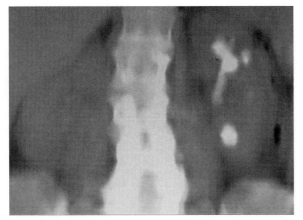

Figure 6.6   A

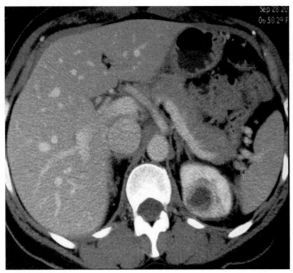

Figure 6.6   C

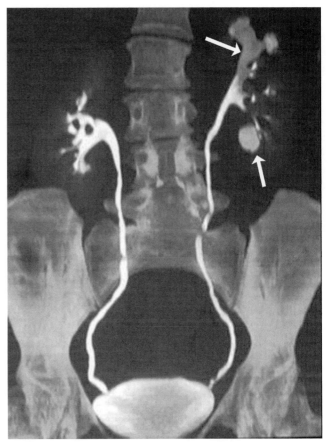

Figure 6.6   B

Findings: Unenhanced coronal average intensity projection image (A) from a CT urogram shows a large branch calculus in the upper pole of the left kidney, a smaller round calculus in the lower pole, and several additional small calculi in the mid kidney. Excretory phase volume-rendered image (B) demonstrates excretion into both renal collecting systems. Calices in the left upper and lower poles are blunted. The calculi in the upper (superior arrow) and lower (inferior arrow) poles can still be seen because they are lower in attenuation than the excreted contrast media. The calcification in the lower pole is located in a caliceal diverticulum. An axial image (C) shows that there is a 3-cm heterogeneous mass in the upper pole of the left kidney, adjacent to the large branch calculus. This mass contains a hypodense center and an evenly thickened wall.

Diagnosis: Left nephrolithiasis and left renal abscess

Discussion: Although some types of urinary tract calculi (e.g., calcium phosphate and magnesium ammonium phosphate stones) may form in chronically infected alkaline urine, urinary tract infection and abscess formation can also be a complication of untreated stone disease, as in this case. When urinary tract infections and stones are concurrent, the infection will often not be treated adequately until the stone, which can serve as an ongoing nidus for infection, has been removed. Many renal abscesses require drainage; however, when the abscesses are small, long-term antibiotic therapy may suffice. (Case courtesy of Richard Cohan, MD, and Elaine Caoili, MD, University of Michigan, Ann Arbor, MI.)

History: 44-year-old paraplegic male, secondary to spine trauma, who developed a severe urinary tract infection. Blood and urine cultures grew *E. coli*.

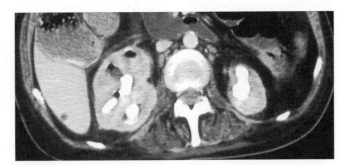

Figure 6.7

Findings: Axial excretory phase image from a CT urogram demonstrates small collections of gas in the right renal collecting system. The left kidney is small, and there is parenchymal scarring—changes that are consistent with chronic pyelonephritis/reflux nephropathy. A small cyst is incidentally identified in the right lobe of the liver.

Diagnosis: Emphysematous pyelitis (see Case 8-18)

Discussion: There are several causes of gas in the renal collecting systems. Gas can be introduced by instrumentation (e.g., retrograde pyelography or ureteroscopy), and by penetrating trauma. Gas introduced via a bladder catheter may reach the renal collecting system in patients with vesicoureteral reflux. Gas may also be found in the collecting system in patients with bowel fistulae. Excluding these causes, gas in the collecting system is the result of a urinary tract infection. When collecting system gas is the sole imaging manifestation of the infection, the process is termed emphysematous pyelitis.

Gas found in the renal parenchyma is called emphysematous pyelonephritis. Gas limited to the perinephric space can be due to a perinephric infection (see Case 6-8). This patient was treated with intravenous antibiotics and recovered completely.

History: 45-year-old diabetic male status post right nephrectomy, with fever and elevated white blood cell count.

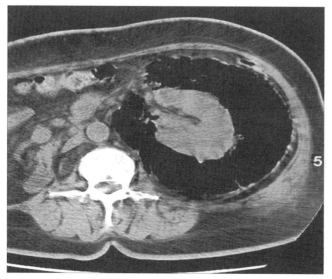

Figure 6.8 A

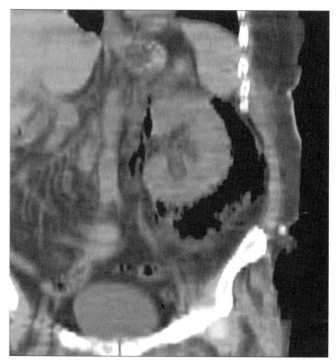

Figure 6.8 B

Findings: Unenhanced axial CT images [axial image (5-mm slice thickness) (A) and coronal image (3-mm slice thickness) (B)] show a large left perinephric collection of gas.

Diagnosis: Gas-producing renal and perinephric infection

Discussion: CT urography can be used to detect gas within and adjacent to the kidney. Emphysematous pyelonephritis is due to renal infection with gas-forming organisms, most commonly *E. coli* and less frequently *Proteus* and *Klebsiella* species. Such an infectious process results in the formation of gas within the renal parenchyma, although gas can also accumulate in the perinephric space. Gas-producing infections are most often seen in patients with diabetes mellitus and have a high mortality, of approximately 40%. Two different types of emphysematous pyelonephritis have been described. In one, focal gas-containing fluid collections can be treated with percutaneous catheter drainage. In the other form, gas is interspersed throughout the renal parenchyma and there is no organized fluid collection. The prognosis is worse in patients without focal, drainable fluid collections. (Case courtesy of Tarek El Diasty, MD, Mansoura University, Mansoura, Egypt.)

CASE 6-9

History: 22-year-old male with brain damage following head trauma developed severe urinary tract infection. Symptoms had not improved following treatment with antibiotics. CT urography was performed to evaluate for urolithiasis and renal abscess.

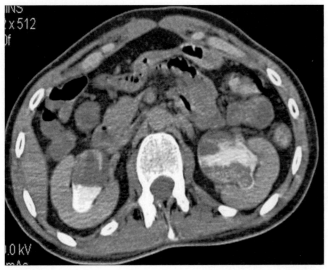

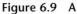

Figure 6.9   A

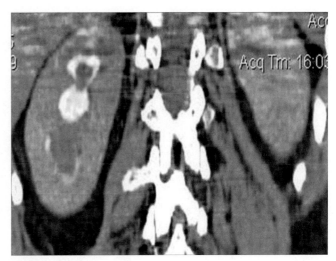

Figure 6.9   B

Findings: Axial (A) and coronal (B) excretory phase images from a CT urogram demonstrate hydronephrosis pelvicaliectasis and extensive debris within both pelvicaliceal systems. The intrarenal collecting system material is noted both anterior and posterior to layering excreted contrast material on the axial images. A discrete filling defect is located in the upper right renal collecting system on the coronal image.

Diagnosis: Acute papillary necrosis associated with urinary tract infection

Discussion: Papillary necrosis is seen most commonly in the setting of chronic diseases such as diabetes mellitus,

sickle cell anemia, analgesic abuse, and chronic urinary tract infection (typically tuberculosis) (see Case 8-5). Rarely, acute renal infection may also cause acute necrotizing papillitis, as in this case. CT urography may be used to demonstrate sloughed papillae in the pelvicaliceal systems and ureters, where they may become lodged and cause obstruction. Sloughed papillae can be suspected on a CT urogram in a patient when blunting of one or more calyces is present in conjunction with contrast material-filled cavities and one or more discrete soft tissue attenuation filling defects in the intrarenal collecting systems or ureters.

CASE 6-10

History: 35-year-old paraplegic male patient with severe kyphoscoliosis secondary to congenital spina bifida and meningomyelocele of the lower thoracic and lumbar spine, and with recurrent urinary tract infections status post urinary diversion and transureteroureterostomy.

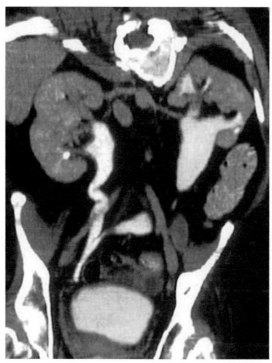

Figure 6.10

Findings: Coronal excretory phase image from a CT urogram demonstrates parenchymal scarring associated with deformity of the adjacent calyces in a small left kidney. There is hypertrophy of normal renal tissue adjacent to the parenchymal scars. Apart from a small cortical scar in its midportion, no abnormalities are seen in the right kidney. The anastomosis of the left-to-right transureteroureterostomy can be seen.

Diagnosis: Chronic pyelonephritis (reflux nephropathy)

Discussion: CT urography can be used to demonstrate the characteristic changes of chronic pyelonephritis (also known as reflux nephropathy) that include renal parenchymal scarring, deformity of adjacent calyces, and reduction in renal size (see Cases 6-10, 7-1, and 8-2). The anatomy of the entire urinary tract, including the anastomosis between the lower part of the left ureter and the right ureter, is also demonstrated on the coronal view. Reflux nephropathy is the result of chronic reflux of infected urine, usually during childhood. As this case demonstrates, the polar regions of the kidneys (particularly the upper poles) are affected more than the interpolar regions because the openings at the level of the papillae in the polar regions are round, which allows for more intrarenal reflux; the openings are slitlike in the interpolar regions of the kidney.

90   *CT Urography: An Atlas*

History: 39-year-old male with dysuria status post treatment with immunosuppressive medications following bone marrow transplantation for chronic myelogenous leukemia.

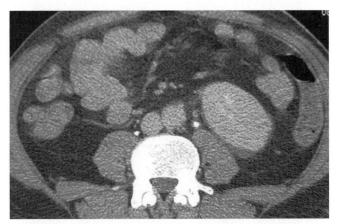

Figure 6.11 A

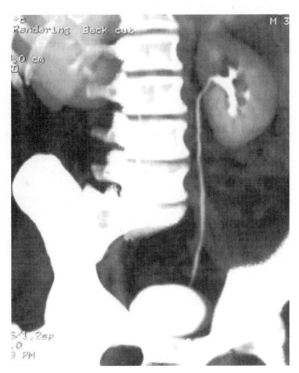

Figure 6.11 C

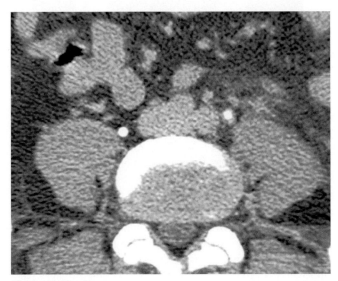

Figure 6.11 B

Findings: Two excretory phase axial images (A, B) obtained at slightly different levels from a CT urogram show moderate circumferential thickening of the left ureteral wall. This process extended from the renal pelvis to the bladder. The ureteral lumen is normal in shape and caliber throughout. This can best be seen on a left posterior oblique excretory phase volume-rendered image (C), in which the left ureter appears normal.

Diagnosis: Acute infectious ureteritis

Discussion: Ureteritis can produce circumferential ureteral wall thickening; however, the differential diagnosis also includes transitional cell carcinoma. Ureteritis can be acute and infectious, as in this patient, or chronic and the result of long-standing irritation and inflammation, as seen in patients with indwelling ureteral stents. CT urography can be used to detect abnormalities of the ureter that involve the wall and periureteral tissues. Prior to CT urography, ureteritis was diagnosed rarely by imaging; IV urography could be used to image predominantly the ureteral lumen. As a result, wall abnormalities could only be detected secondarily. Volume-rendered images are similar to IV urography; only the lumen is demonstrated, and therefore the findings of ureteritis are not demonstrated. (Case courtesy of Richard Cohan, MD, and Elaine Caoili, MD, University of Michigan, Ann Arbor, MI.)

History: 55-year-old male with pyuria and history of long-standing recurrent urinary tract infections.

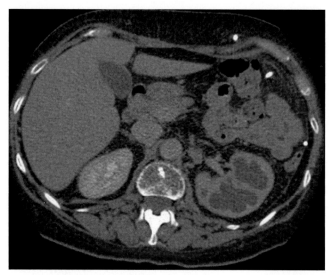

Figure 6.12 A

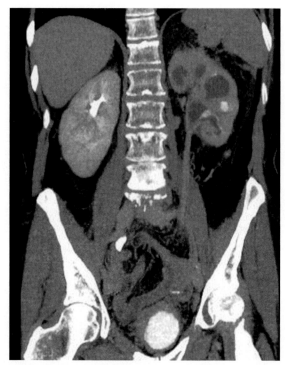

Figure 6.12 B

Findings: Axial CT image (A) demonstrates large areas of low attenuation within the central portion of the left kidney. On a coronal reformatted image (B), the low attenuation can be identified as corresponding to a dilated left renal collecting system. The wall of the left ureter is thickened throughout its length, and there is inflammatory stranding in the peri-ureteral fat. High attenuation material in the left kidney represents calcification.

Diagnosis: Renal and ureteral tuberculosis

Discussion: Genitourinary tuberculosis develops due to hematogenous seeding of the kidneys, usually from an infection that originated in the lungs. The kidneys are nearly always affected prior to other parts of the urinary tract. One of the early findings in renal tuberculosis is papillary necrosis. Over time, renal parenchymal calcifications develop in up to 50% of patients. The kidneys may become scarred. Subsequently, the inflammatory process may spread to the collecting systems and ureters. Urinary tract tuberculosis then produces abnormal peristalsis, ureteral wall thickening, and strictures, with dilatation proximal to the strictures. Ureteral wall thickening can be more easily identified at CT urography using cross-sectional images than at intravenous urography or on volume-rendered images since the latter depict only the urinary tract lumen. In this patient, the ureter is diffusely involved. Hydronephrosis is likely due to abnormal peristalsis and mild obstruction resulting from ureteral involvement. (Case courtesy of Nigel Cowan, MD, Oxford University, Oxford, UK.)

History: A 65-year-old male with a history of tuberculosis of the urinary tract presents with urinary frequency and dysuria.

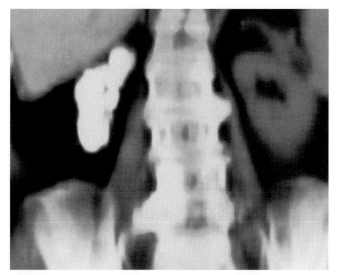

Figure 6.13   A

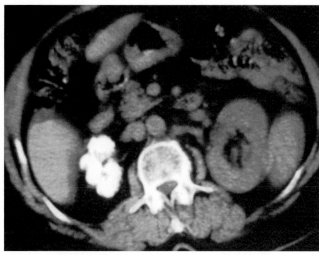

Figure 6.13   B

Findings: Unenhanced coronal (A) and axial (B) images of the upper abdomen demonstrate extensive calcification forming a cast of the entire right kidney. No viable right renal parenchyma is identified. No significant abnormality is seen in the left kidney.

Diagnosis: Tuberculosis of the right kidney (auto-nephrectomy)

Discussion: Stricture formation at sites of normal anatomical narrowing (the infundibula, ureteropelvic junction, and ureterovesical junction) is a characteristic complication of tuberculosis (TB) of the urinary tract. Although the patient in this case was examined with unenhanced CT alone, CT urography can be used to detect abnormalities of the urinary tract secondary to TB. Loss of definition of the affected minor calyx (the so-called "moth-eaten appearance") and irregularities and a nodular appearance of the ureteral wall may be seen at the early stages of the infection. Long-term manifestations include caliectasis proximal to infundibular strictures. A dilated calyx may fail to opacify during excretory phase images if an infundibular stenosis is severe and the resulting obstruction high-grade. Tuberculous abscesses may develop and be observed as low-attenuation areas on unenhanced and nephrographic phase images, and they may or may not contain opacified urine on delayed excretory phase images (depending on whether or not they have excavated into the renal collecting systems). Destruction of the renal parenchyma and fibrosis may produce appearances identical to those seen in nontuberculous chronic pyelonephritis. In long-standing cases, caseating material in dilated calyces may calcify and produce a cast of the pelvicaliceal system. This is referred to as autonephrectomy, as shown in this case. Other patterns of renal calcification may also be seen, including irregular and ill-defined calcifications in the renal parenchyma or curvilinear calcifications mimicking the type of calcification that can be seen occasionally in benign complicated renal cysts. (Case courtesy of Tarek El Diasty, MD, Mansoura University, Mansoura, Egypt.)

History: 46-year-old paraplegic male (secondary to spinal injury) with a history of recurrent urinary tract infections and renal stones.

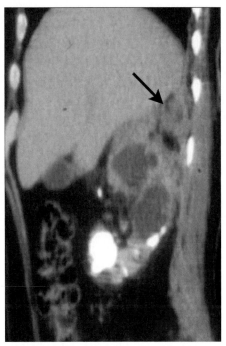

Figure 6.14   A

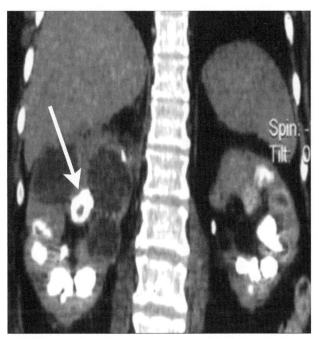

Figure 6.14   B

Findings: Sagittal (A) and coronal (B) excretory phase images from a CT urogram show severe caliectasis in the upper pole of the right kidney, which does not contain any excreted contrast material. There is a large high-attenuation focus (white arrow) with a low-attenuation area in its center in the midportion of the right kidney, which represents an obstructing calculus, impacted in an infundibulum. Dilated calyces filled with contrast medium are seen in the lower pole of the right kidney as well as in the left kidney, the latter also being small in size and associated with parenchymal scarring. In addition, there is a poorly defined, heterogeneous, 3-cm mass (black arrow) extending from the upper pole of the right kidney into the posterior abdominal wall. This mass contains several areas of low attenuation.

Diagnosis: Xanthogranulomatous pyelonephritis

Discussion: Xanthogranulomatous pyelonephritis is an uncommon complication of renal infection (see Cases 5-15 and 8-19). It is more common in females. It is also more often seen in diabetics and in the majority of cases arises as a complication of long-standing urinary tract obstruction and stones. A variety of infecting organisms can be found, with *Proteus* species and *E. coli* being most frequent. On pathology, xanthogranulomatous pyelonephritis has a distinctive appearance; the inflammatory process contains granulomatous areas composed of histiocytes with foamy fat-containing cytoplasm. These are called xanthoma cells, thus explaining the origin of this disease's name. Xanthogranulomatous pyelonephritis is most commonly a diffuse process, affecting an entire kidney. When the entire kidney is involved, there is usually no normal functioning renal parenchyma. The inflamed tissue may enhance. On images obtained at CT urography, large areas of low attenuation, representing pus and debris, often surround a large, chronically obstructing, staghorn or branch calculus. The affected kidney is typically enlarged but preserves its normal reniform shape. The inflammatory process may extend into the perinephric tissue. Perinephric stranding is usually seen, but there may also be perinephric inflammatory masses or abscesses, as in this patient. Less commonly, xanthogranulomatous pyelonephritis may manifest as a focal inflammatory mass and affect only a portion of a kidney. Focal or segmental xanthogranulomatous pyelonephritis may also be caused by an obstructing calculus with ongoing infection and may spread into adjacent perinephric tissues. Focal xanthogranulomatous pyelonephritis may occur without calculi. In these patients, focal xanthogranulomatous pyelonephritis can have an appearance similar to renal cancer. Treatment includes percutaneous drainage of perinephric fluid collections. When diffuse disease is present, nephrectomy is usually performed. In comparison, partial nephrectomy may suffice in patients with the focal form of the disease. There are reports of focal xanthogranulomatous pyelonephritis being successfully treated with antibiotics alone.

CASE 6-15

History: 50-year-old diabetic female with chronic renal insufficiency presents with failure to thrive, frequency, and dysuria.

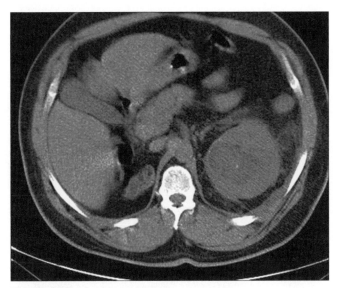

Figure 6.15 A

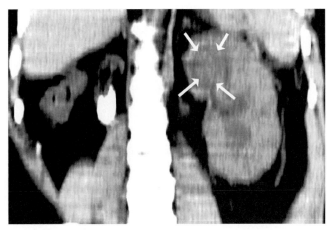

Figure 6.15 B

Findings: Axial (A) and coronal unenhanced CT (B) images of the upper abdomen show left hydronephrosis with the attenuation of the dilated left renal calyces being higher than water. The coronal image (B) demonstrates a round soft tissue attenuation mass (arrows) surrounded by urine in the upper pole calices. The axial image (A) also shows a punctate high-attenuation central focus within the soft tissue mass. The right kidney is atrophic and there is a large stone in its lower pole (B).

Diagnosis: Candidal infection of the left kidney

Discussion: Fungal infection of the urinary tract is most often seen in immunocompromised patients, particularly diabetics, IV drug abusers, patients with AIDS, and other patients who are immunosuppressed. Candida, aspergillus, mucor, coccidioides, cryptococcus, actinomyces, and nocardia are common fungi that infect the urinary tract. They can cause acute pyelonephritis, papillary necrosis, and multiple intrarenal and perinephric abscesses. Fungus balls, which consist of concretions of fungal material, may form in the pelvicaliceal system and cause obstruction. Fungus balls appear as filling defects on images obtained at CT urography and occasionally can be seen on unenhanced images, as in this case. Fungus balls have a higher attenuation than water. They can also be demonstrated with antegrade pyelography, as was subsequently performed in this patient prior to nephrostomy. In this case, the fungus balls were removed percutaneously. (Case courtesy of Tarek El Diasty, MD, Mansoura University, Mansoura, Egypt.)

History: 50-year-old male with a history of urinary tract schistosomiasis, with known right ureteral stricture, now presents with right flank pain.

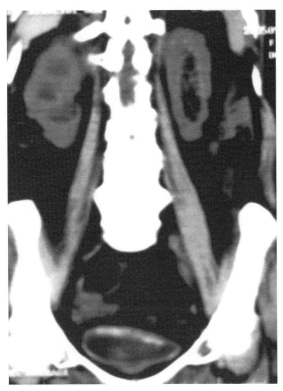

Figure 6.16 A

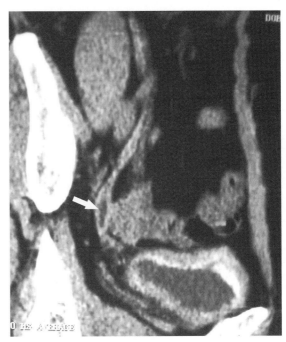

Figure 6.16 B

Findings: Coronal (A) and coronal oblique (B) images demonstrate calcification of the bladder and lower third of the right ureter (arrow) associated with right-sided hydronephrosis. No urinary tract calculi are identified. There is left renal parenchymal scarring.

Diagnosis: Urinary schistosomiasis

Discussion: Schistosomiasis primarily affects the urinary bladder and lower thirds of the ureters. Isolated renal involvement is rare. However, renal complications secondary to schistosomiasis of the lower urinary tract may occur and include acute pyelonephritis, reflux nephropathy, obstructive nephropathy, stone formation, schistosomiasis-associated glomerulonephritis, and amyloidosis. Early in the disease, schistosomiasis causes edema of the bladder mucosa, which can produce small filling defects in the bladder. Similar small nodular filling defects may also be seen in the ureters. Later in the disease, calcifications appear in the bladder wall. Ureteral calcifications are less common but, when present, can affect the entire ureter. Ureteral calcifications are found typically in the submucosa but may also be found in the muscle and serosa. Ureteral dilatation and tortuosity may occur even in the absence of obstruction. Ureteral strictures are often located in the lower or intravesical portions of the ureter. Ureteral calculi are also common and usually situated proximal to strictures. Squamous cell carcinoma of the urinary bladder is a common long-term complication of ongoing urinary tract schistosomiasis. Findings associated with schistosomiasis of the urinary tract may be depicted with CT urography. Unenhanced images are especially important in assessing calcifications in the bladder and ureter and for detecting stones. (Case courtesy of Tarek El Diasty, MD, Mansoura University, Mansoura, Egypt.)

SUGGESTED READINGS

1. Baumgarten DA, Baumgartner BR. Imaging and radiologic management of upper urinary tract infections. *Urol Clin North Am.* 1997;24:545–569.

2. Benson M, Li Puma JP, Resnick MI. The role of imaging studies in urinary tract infection. *Urol Clin North Am.* 1986;13:605–625.

3. Browne RF, Zwirewich C, Torreggiani WC. Imaging of urinary tract infection in the adult. *Eur Radiol.* 2004;14(Suppl 3):168–183.

4. Gold RP, McLennan BL. Renal inflammation. In: Pollack HM, McLennan BL, Dyer R, et al., eds. *Clinical urography.* Philadelphia: Saunders; 2000:923–947.

5. Kawashima A, Sandler CM, Goldman SM. Imaging in acute renal infection. *BJU Int.* 2000;86(Suppl 1):70–79.

6. Kawashima A, LeRoy AJ. Radiologic evaluation of patients with renal infections. *Infect Dis Clin North Am.* 2003;17:433–456.

7. Soulen MC, Fishman EK, Goldman SM, et al. Bacterial renal infection: role of CT. *Radiology.* 1989;171:703–707.

8. Talner LB, Davidson AJ, Lebowitz RL, et al. Acute pyelonephritis: can we agree on terminology? *Radiology.* 1994;192:297–305.

CHAPTER SEVEN
RENAL MASSES

Lisa M. Zorn, MD

Stuart G. Silverman, MD

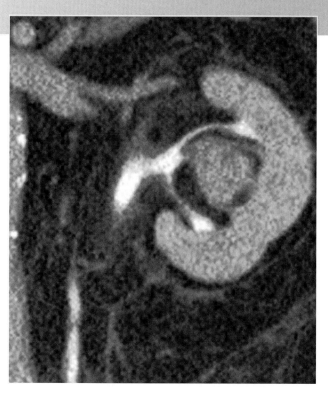

CASE 7-1

History: 33-year-old female with a history of nephrolithiasis and left flank pain.

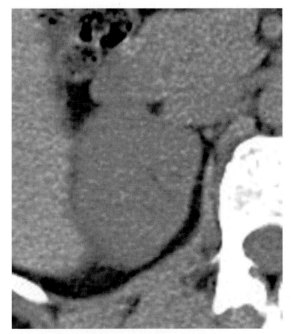

Figure 7.1   A

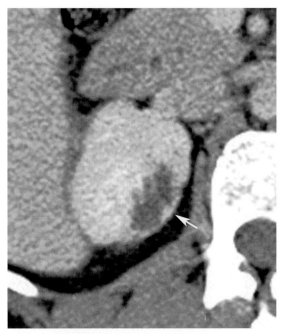

Figure 7.1   B

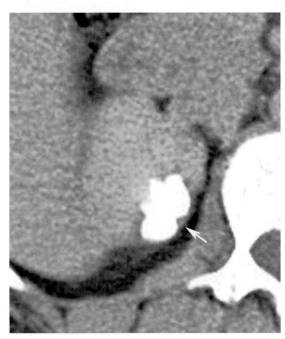

Figure 7.1   C

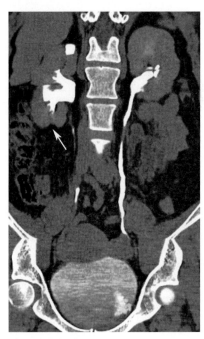

Figure 7.1   D

Findings: Axial unenhanced (A) and nephrographic (B) images from a CT urogram demonstrate a 2.5 × 1.6 × 1.5 cm, low-attenuation cystic mass with lobulated margins in the upper pole of the right kidney. Nephrographic phase image (B) demonstrates thin septations and an enhancing outer wall (arrow). Axial image in the excretory phase (C) shows that the lesion fills with contrast material (arrow). Coronal image (D) demonstrates multiple areas of focal parenchymal scarring (arrow) at the superior and inferior poles of both kidneys along with caliectasis.

Diagnosis: Reflux nephropathy

Discussion: The process of progressive renal injury with associated reflux of infected urine is called reflux nephropathy (see Cases 6-10 and 8-2). Intrarenal reflux of infected urine damages the affected renal lobe, resulting in caliectasis and associated parenchymal scarring. Reflux nephropathy affects the polar regions of the kidneys preferentially. CT urography was helpful in this case by providing excretory phase images and coronal displays. The upper pole abnormality may have been mistaken for a cystic neoplasm if the excretory phase was not included. Coronal displays are valuable in noting that the poles are affected preferentially. Also, coronal images can be used to confirm that the caliectasis is associated with renal scarring.

History: 67-year-old female with hydronephrosis.

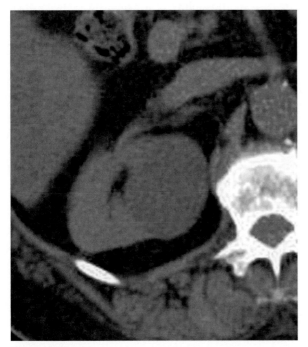

Figure 7.2   A

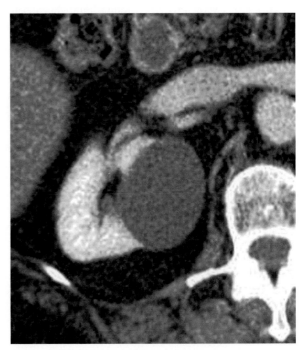

Figure 7.2   B

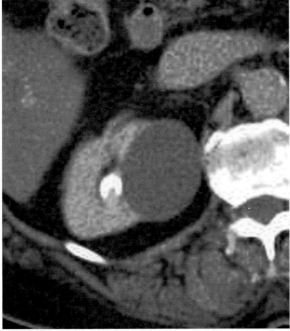

Figure 7.2   C

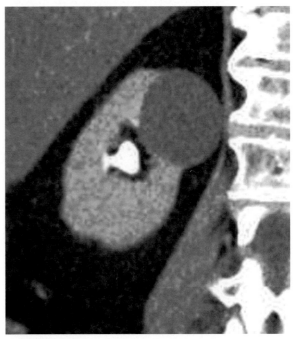

Figure 7.2   D

Findings: Axial unenhanced (A), nephrographic (B), and excretory phase (C) images and coronal excretory phase (D) images from a CT urogram demonstrate a homogeneous, low-attenuation, 4-cm mass in the upper pole of the right kidney. The mass has a smooth, thin wall, contains no septations or calcifications, and does not enhance.

Diagnosis: Simple renal cyst

Discussion: Simple renal cyst is the most common renal mass and is thought to arise from tubular obstruction, renal vascular compromise, or medullary interstitial fibrosis. They are found in half the population older than age 50 years. Simple cysts are often multiple and bilateral. Small cysts are almost always asymptomatic. Large cysts may cause obstruction, pain, hematuria, or hypertension. In order to be diagnosed as a simple cyst, a mass should be well-marginated, low attenuation (<20 HU), contain no septations or calcifications, and be nonenhancing (i.e., the mass should not enhance by more than 10 HU after contrast material administration). Simple renal cysts are classified by Bosniak as category I cysts and can be diagnosed definitively as benign. CT urography with thin sections provides a detailed search of renal cysts for complicating features that might raise the possibility of a malignant cystic neoplasm. Thin section images can also be used to reduce partial volume averaging. As a result, attenuation measurements of renal masses can be obtained with more confidence. In general, attenuation measurements of a renal mass can be considered accurate only if the mass's diameter is at least twice the image section thickness. For example, cysts as small as 6 mm may be characterized confidently with a CT urography protocol that includes 3-mm sections before and after contrast media administration but would likely not be measured accurately if 5-mm-thick sections had been obtained. Simple renal cysts can be differentiated from caliectasis as a result of reflux nephropathy (see Case 7-1), peripelvic cysts (see Case 7-4), and calyceal diverticula (see Case 7-5) by examining the excretory phase images obtained with CT urography because on excretory phase images, caliectasis and calyceal diverticula usually contain opacified urine, whereas renal cysts do not.

History: 60-year-old female with left flank pain and left renal mass.

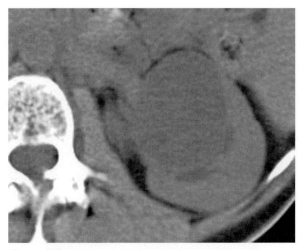

Figure 7.3   A

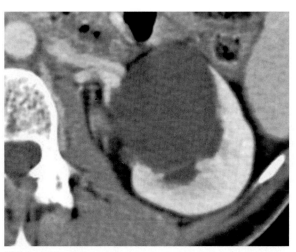

Figure 7.3   B

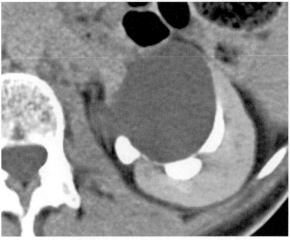

Figure 7.3   C

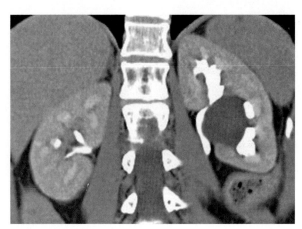

Figure 7.3   D

Findings: Axial unenhanced (A), nephrographic (B), and excretory (C) images from a CT urogram demonstrate a nonenhancing, low-attenuation, well-marginated, 4-cm cystic mass in the left kidney without septations or calcifications. Coronal image (D) shows mild hydronephrosis.

Diagnosis: Parapelvic cyst

Discussion: This mass fulfills all the CT-based criteria for a simple cyst. Approximately half of the cyst's circumference is surrounded by renal parenchyma. This "claw sign" indicates that the cyst arises from the kidney. Since the cyst abuts the renal sinus and arises from the kidney, it is called a parapelvic cyst. Parapelvic cysts are typically solitary masses that may contain low-level echoes on sonography. Peripelvic cysts are typically multiple, often bilateral, and smaller than parapelvic cysts (see Case 7-4). Because of their central location, parapelvic cysts may cause mild obstruction of the infundibula and calyces. Cystic masses that are located in or around the renal hilum cannot be differentiated from the intrarenal collecting system on unenhanced and nephrographic phase images. Excretory phase images are needed to differentiate the collecting system (which in many cases contains opacified urine) from cystic masses (which do not).

CASE 7-4

History: 52-year-old female with gross hematuria.

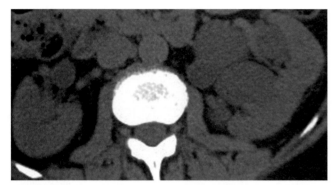

Figure 7.4 A

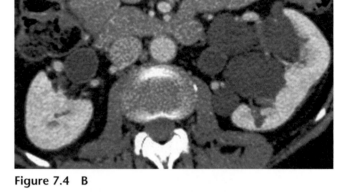

Figure 7.4 B

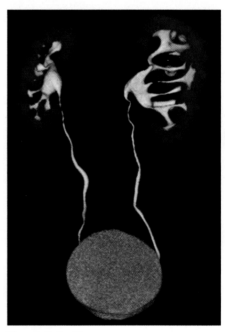

Figure 7.4 C

Figure 7.4 D

Findings: Axial unenhanced (A) and nephrographic phase (B) images show multiple, well-marginated, low-attenuation (<20 HU), nonenhancing masses in the renal sinus of the left kidney. A small (<1 cm), low-attenuation lesion in the renal parenchyma is almost certainly a cyst. Coronal reformatted image during the excretory phase (C) reveals the intrarenal collecting system filled with contrast material and demonstrates cystic masses on both sides of most infundibula. Volume-rendered image (D) does not directly display the cysts but, rather, their compressive effects on the attenuated adjacent opacified intrarenal collecting system.

Diagnosis: Peripelvic cysts

Discussion: Peripelvic cysts originate from renal sinus structures and insinuate themselves in the sinus fat. They are thought to be lymphatic in origin. This condition may also be referred to as congenital renal pelvic lymphangiectasia.

In contrast, parapelvic cysts arise from renal parenchyma and expand into the renal sinus (see Case 7-3). Peripelvic cysts are common and usually multiple. They frequently distort the calyces and can attenuate and stretch the infundibula. Peripelvic cysts mimic hydronephrosis on ultrasound. CT urography displays the relation of the renal sinus cysts to the adjacent intrarenal collecting system. Peripelvic cysts can be difficult to distinguish from hydronephrosis on CT scans in which only unenhanced, corticomedullary, or nephrographic phase scans are obtained. CT urography, specifically the excretory phase images in the coronal plane, displays all components of the collecting system and shows how the infundibula and calyces are splayed by the cysts. If only volume-rendered images are utilized, as with excretory urography, the differential diagnosis would include peripelvic cysts and renal sinus lipomatosis.

History: 28-year-old female with urinary frequency.

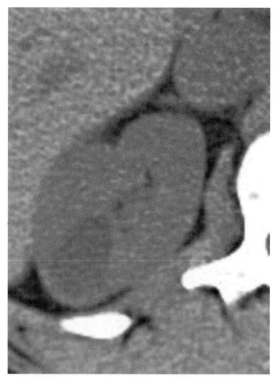

Figure 7.5   A

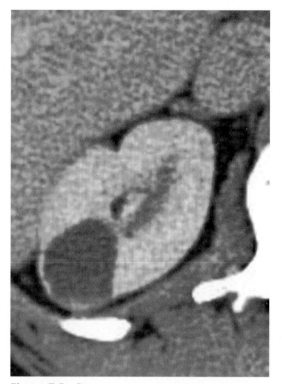

Figure 7.5   B

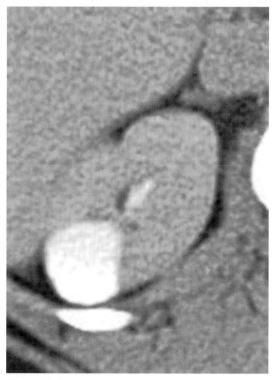

Figure 7.5   C

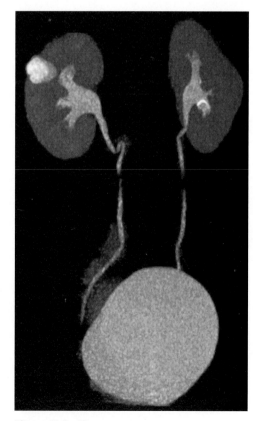

Figure 7.5   D

Findings: Axial unenhanced (A) and nephrographic (B) images from a CT urogram demonstrate a well-marginated, low-attenuation, nonenhancing, 2.5-cm cystic mass in the upper pole of the right kidney without septations or calcifications. The lesion fills with contrast material during the excretory phase (C). Maximum intensity projection image during the excretory phase (D) demonstrates a collection of contrast material situated lateral to an upper pole calyx.

Diagnosis: Congenital calyceal diverticulum

Discussion: Calyceal diverticula are congenital lesions that occur when one of the last generation of tubules in the first period of dichotomous division fails to expand as it normally would to form the infundibulum of a minor calyx and remains as a diverticulum (see Cases 4-13 and 8-4). Calyceal diverticula are lined by uroepithelium and communicate through a thin channel with the fornix of a calyx. They are usually asymptomatic, particularly when small. Calculi may develop and cause pain in large diverticula. Infection may also develop. A calyceal diverticulum may mimic a renal cyst or neoplasm if excretory phase images are not obtained. Calyceal diverticula usually fill with contrast material on excretory phase images; renal cysts and neoplasms almost always do not. The differential diagnosis on CT urography also includes residual abscess cavities and cysts that communicate with the collecting system.

CASE 7-6

History: 57-year-old male with hematuria.

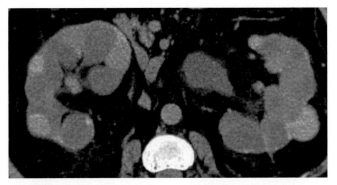

Figure 7.6   A

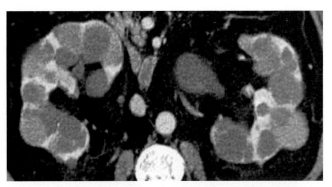

Figure 7.6   B

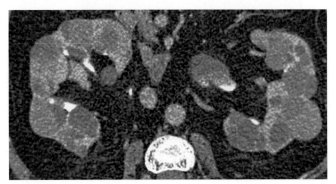

Figure 7.6   C

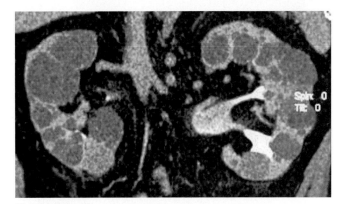

Figure 7.6   D

Findings: Axial unenhanced (A), nephrographic (B), and excretory (C) images show that both kidneys are enlarged and contain innumerable parenchymal cystic masses of varying sizes. Coronal reformatted image in the excretory phase (D) shows that the kidneys are also enlarged in the cephalocaudal dimension (14.0 cm on the right; 14.5 cm on the left). On the unenhanced image (A), some cysts are hyperdense (more dense than renal parenchyma). When each cystic mass's attenuation was measured on both unenhanced and enhanced images, none enhanced.

Diagnosis: Autosomal dominant polycystic kidney disease

Discussion: Autosomal dominant (adult) polycystic kidney disease is a hereditary disorder that usually manifests clinically in the third or fourth decade of life with hypertension, hematuria, or renal failure. Renal cysts develop as the patient ages, eventually completely replacing the renal parenchyma. Their appearance as innumerable, low-attenuation lesions at the nephrographic phase on intravenous urograms has been described as the "Swiss cheese" nephrogram, a term that also aptly describes their appearance on CT urography. Hemorrhage within some of the cysts results in their hyperdense appearance on CT. The cysts may also cause pain or become infected. Patients typically develop cysts in other organs, such as the liver (70%), pancreas (10%), spleen (5%), and, rarely, the ovary and thyroid. Intracranial berry aneurysms develop in 20% of patients. End-stage renal disease occurs in 45% of patients with autosomal dominant polycystic kidney disease by the age of 60 years.

History: 52-year-old male with urinary incontinence and retention and an incidentally detected cystic renal mass on ultrasound.

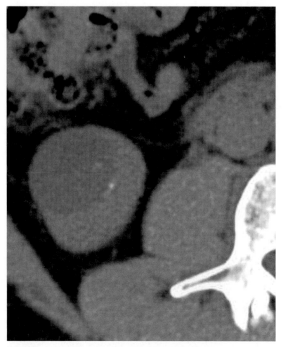

Figure 7.7   A

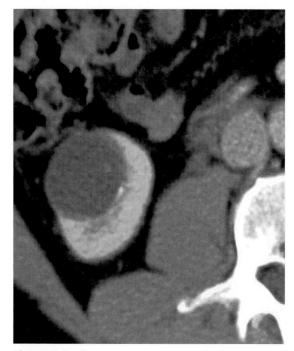

Figure 7.7   B

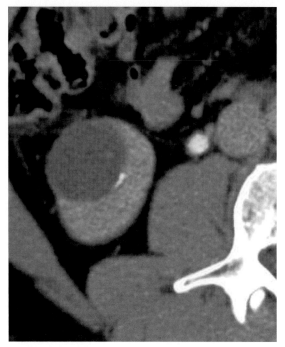

Figure 7.7   C

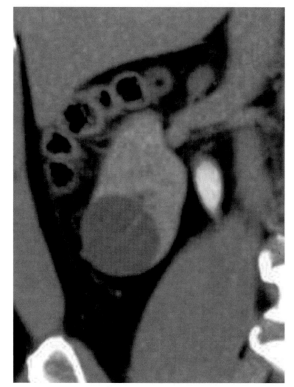

Figure 7.7   D

Findings: Axial unenhanced (A), nephrographic (B), and excretory (C) phase images from a CT urogram demonstrate a 3.8-cm, low-attenuation mass in the lower pole of the right kidney that contains a thin septation and thin calcifications in both the septation and the medial wall of the mass (A). Coronal excretory phase image (D) demonstrates that the septation is thin and enhancing, as evidenced by the fact that the septation is seen more clearly with contrast media than without it.

Diagnosis: Benign, complicated renal cyst

Discussion: Cystic renal masses that contain few (<3), thin (1 or 2 mm) septations are classified as Bosniak category II cystic masses. Calcifications may be present, as long as they are small and border forming (i.e., located in the wall or septation). Bosniak category II cystic masses, which also include hyperdense cysts (see Case 7-8), are reliably considered benign on imaging findings alone. Renal masses that contain more thin septations, thick or nodular calcifications, or those masses that fulfill the criteria for a hyperdense cyst but are >3 cm or intrarenal are considered Bosniak category IIF lesions. These masses are usually benign but should be followed. The "F" refers to the need for follow-up imaging. CT urography provides thin section evaluation of the mass's features before and after contrast media administration.

History: 46-year-old female with an incidental renal mass.

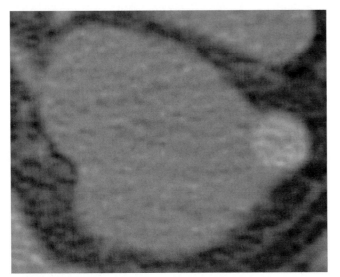

Figure 7.8   A

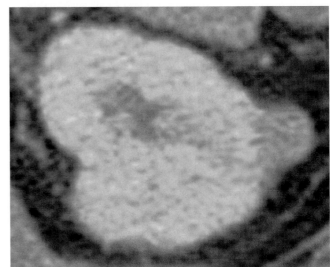

Figure 7.8   B

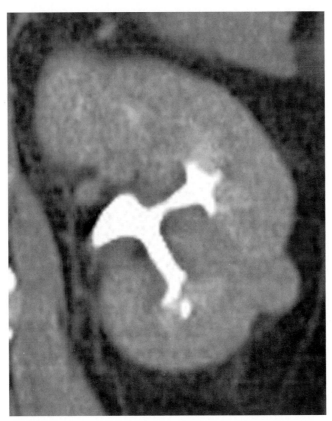

Figure 7.8   C

Findings: Axial unenhanced (A) and nephrographic phase (B) images from a CT urogram demonstrate a 1.1-cm, homogenously hyperdense (70 HU), exophytic mass in the lateral aspect of the lower pole of the left kidney. Nephrographic phase image demonstrates that the mass's attenuation remains the same (70 HU); therefore, the mass does not enhance. Coronal excretory phase image obtained at 15 minutes after contrast media administration (C) also demonstrates that the mass's attenuation is unchanged.

Diagnosis: Benign, hyperdense renal cyst

Discussion: Renal masses that are denser than renal parenchyma (i.e., >40 HU) are considered hyperdense and usually measure 50 to 90 HU. Most hyperdense renal masses are benign hyperdense cysts, as in this case. These cysts, as in Case 7-7, are classified as Bosniak category II cysts and are likely benign. However, a diagnosis of a benign, hyperdense cyst requires all the following criteria to be fulfilled: the mass must be small (≤3 cm), homogeneously hyperdense (even using a narrow window setting), well-marginated, nonenhancing, and have at least one-fourth of its circumference extend outside the renal parenchyma so a portion of its wall can be evaluated. A high concentration of protein or blood breakdown products is responsible for their high attenuation. If a hyperdense mass is noted on an enhanced CT alone and the study is being monitored, 15-minute delayed CT can be performed to determine the presence of wash-out of contrast media or "de-enhancement." If the mass de-enhances, the mass can be considered solid and neoplastic (excluding vascular abnormalities). However, if the mass does not de-enhance, it can be reliably considered a benign, hyperdense cyst.

History: 42-year-old asymptomatic male potential kidney donor.

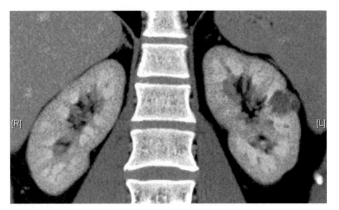

Figure 7.9   A

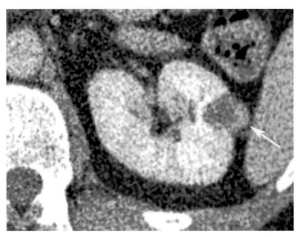

Figure 7.9   B

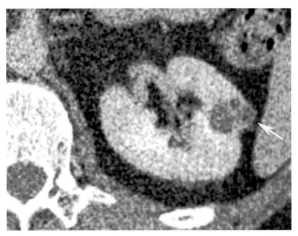

Figure 7.9   C

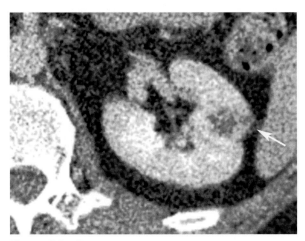

Figure 7.9   D

Findings: Coronal image during the nephrographic phase (A) shows a 2.5 × 1.6-cm septated cystic mass in the interpolar region of the left kidney. This image is a 3-mm-thick section obtained from 2.5-mm collimated data. Axial nephrographic phase images reconstructed in 3-mm sections at 1.5-mm increments (B–D) demonstrate that some of the septations are thick and nodular (arrows).

Diagnosis: Cystic renal cell carcinoma, clear cell type

Discussion: The differential diagnosis of a multiseptated cystic renal mass includes multilocular cyst, multilocular cystic nephroma, and multilocular cystic renal cell carcinoma. Multiseptated cystic masses that contain thick septations are indeterminate for malignancy and included in Bosniak's category III. Since both benign and malignant lesions can have this appearance, these masses are generally resected surgically. Cystic masses that contain nodular enhancement have a high probability of malignancy and are included in Bosniak's category IV. When this mass was imaged using 5-mm-thick sections (A), the septations appeared thin and the presence of nodular enhancement was questionable. The mass was initially considered a Bosniak category III lesion. In comparison, when the mass was imaged using 3-mm sections and 1.5-mm increments, the mass was clearly shown to have thick septations and nodular components and was therefore reclassified as a Bosniak category IV cyst. This case exemplifies the importance of evaluating all renal masses thoroughly with thin section images so as to detect subtle enhancing nodules. This case also shows how CT urography, performed with an MDCT scanner, can be used to provide a detailed search of cystic renal masses. "Ultra-thin" section CT (3 mm-thick sections) can be obtained using collimations that are 2.5 mm or less. Reconstructing thinly collimated data as thin section images does not increase radiation dose to the patient. However, it does increase the number of images that need to be evaluated.

CASE 7-10

History: 37-year-old female with an incidental finding.

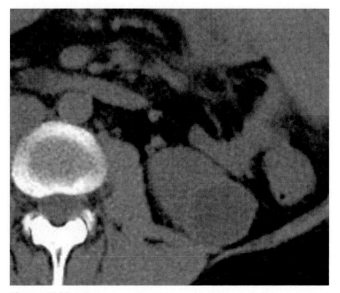

Figure 7.10　A

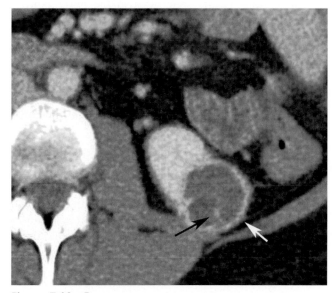

Figure 7.10　B

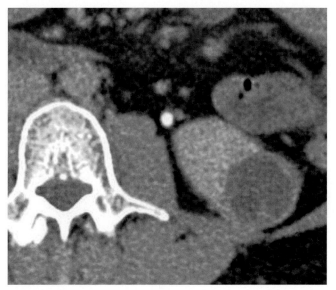

Figure 7.10　C

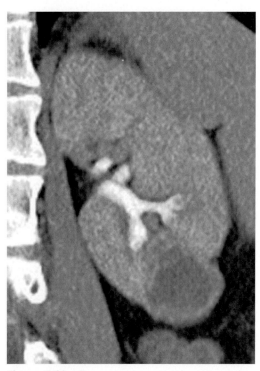

Figure 7.10　D

Findings: Axial unenhanced (A), nephrographic (B), and excretory phase (C) images from a CT urogram demonstrate a 3-cm multiloculated cystic mass in the lower pole of the left kidney. The posterior wall and the septations are thickened and enhance by more than 20 HU. Hounsfield measurements of the wall (white arrow) are 25 HU on unenhanced, 77 HU on nephrographic, and 54 HU on excretory phase. A septum (black arrow) enhances from 8 HU on unenhanced phase to 31 HU on nephrographic phase. The coronal images (D) demonstrate thick walls and show that the mass is partially exophytic.

Diagnosis: Cystic renal cell carcinoma, clear cell type

Discussion: Multilocular cystic masses may represent benign multilocular cysts, multilocular cystic nephroma, or multilocular renal cell carcinoma. Since both benign and malignant causes are included in the differential diagnosis, masses with this appearance are considered indeterminate and categorized as Bosniak category III lesions. Many masses with this appearance are ultimately diagnosed as renal cancers. Therefore, Bosniak category III cysts are considered surgical lesions. When encountering a multiloculated cystic mass, the presence of enhancing, thickened walls and septations (best seen on the nephrographic phase images in this case) increases the chance that a mass is malignant. Masses that enhance by more than 10 HU are considered enhancing, particularly if they enhance by more than 20 HU. CT urography includes both unenhanced and enhanced images so that enhancement may be detected. Thin section images are obtained so that septations may be discerned in detail and analyzed accurately for enhancement (see Case 7-9). In addition to axial images, data acquired at CT urography can be used to visualize renal masses and their relationship to renal collecting systems and blood vessels in sagittal, coronal, and oblique planes.

CASE 7-11

History: 36-year-old female with nausea and abdominal pain.

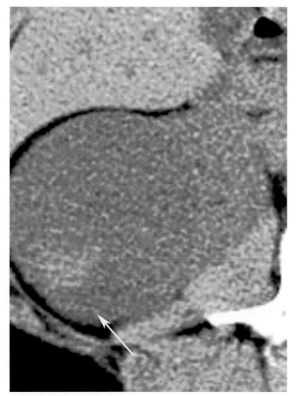

Figure 7.11   A

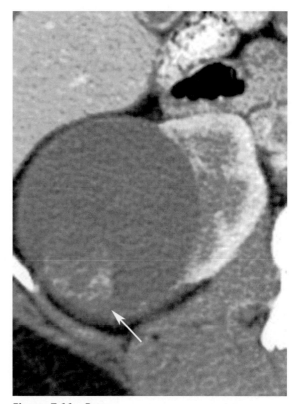

Figure 7.11   B

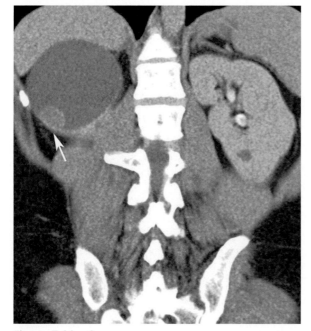

Figure 7.11   C

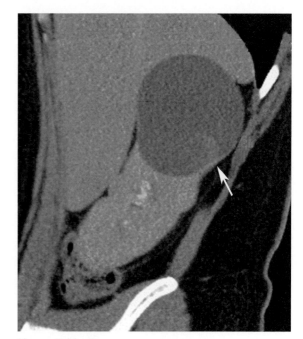

Figure 7.11   D

Findings: Axial unenhanced (A) and corticomedullary phase (B) images as well as coronal (C) and sagittal (D) excretory phase images from a CT urogram demonstrate an 8-cm cystic mass in the upper pole of the right kidney with a solitary enhancing nodule (arrows) in the infero-posterior aspect of what otherwise appears as a benign cyst. The nodular component measures 50 HU on the unenhanced image (A) and 70 HU on the corticomedullary phase image (B).

Diagnosis: Multilocular cystic renal cell carcinoma, clear cell type

Discussion: Cystic renal masses that contain enhancing nodules are included in Bosniak's category IV. The probability of renal cell carcinoma is high because the nodular components at pathology almost always represent islands of tumor. CT urography protocols that include thin sections help detect small areas of nodular enhancement (see Case 7-9). This case also demonstrates the value of multiplanar reconstructions that help detect enhancing tumor nodules and differentiate them from those apparent nodules that are caused by partial volume averaging with adjacent enhancing renal parenchyma.

History: 41-year-old male with hematuria.

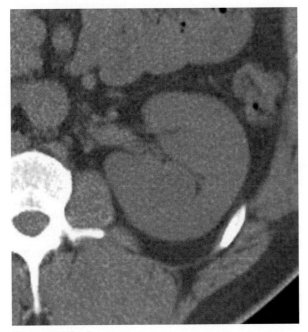

Figure 7.12   A

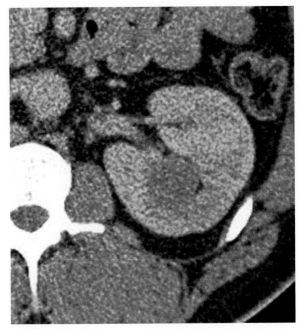

Figure 7.12   B

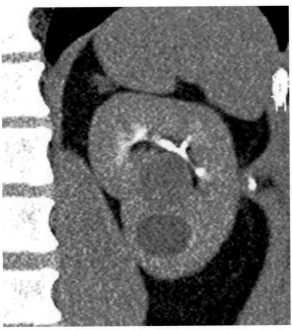

Figure 7.12   C

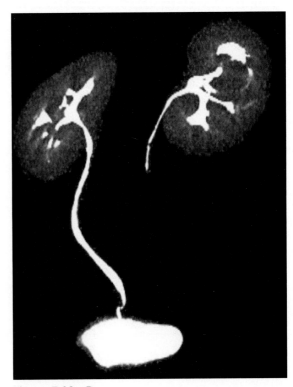

Figure 7.12   D

Findings: Axial unenhanced (A) and nephrographic phase (B) images demonstrate a 3-cm mass in the lower pole of the left kidney. The mass measures 21 HU before and 35 HU after contrast material administration. Coronal excretory image (C) also shows a simple cyst inferior to the mass. Maximum intensity projection image (D) demonstrates the relationship of the mass to the collecting system.

Diagnosis: Renal cell carcinoma, papillary type

Discussion: CT urography should include images of the kidneys before and after IV contrast material so that renal masses may be evaluated for the presence of fat, calcifications, and contrast material enhancement. Excluding inflammatory causes and vascular abnormalities, small, solitary renal masses that homogeneously enhance are solid neoplasms. The most common renal neoplasms include renal cell carcinoma (see Case 7-14), oncocytoma (see Case 7-15), angiomyolipoma (see Case 7-18), metastasis, and lymphoma. Transitional cell carcinoma (see Case 7-16) may also present as a solid renal mass. Renal cell carcinoma is the most common malignant renal neoplasm. Hemorrhage and necrosis occur commonly in these tumors, so renal cell carcinoma may appear as partially or even predominantly cystic or multiloculated. The solid components of these tumors are often hypervascular. Tumor invasion into the renal vein and inferior vena cava occurs in 30% and 5% to 10% of cases, respectively. Papillary renal cancers are the second most common type of renal cell carcinoma, affecting approximately 10% to 15% of patients. Papillary renal cell carcinoma may occur sporadically or as a hereditary disease presenting in family members as multifocal tumor nodules in both kidneys. Papillary renal cell carcinomas are hypovascular neoplasms that usually enhance, but typically only mildly (approximately 20 HU), as in this case (14 HU). Three-dimensional images may help with surgical planning; the maximum intensity projection image in this case showed that the mass was located close to the upper pole intrarenal collecting system.

History: 71-year-old male with anemia and familial history of colon cancer.

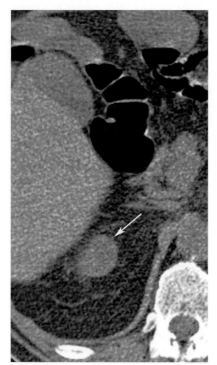

Figure 7.13   A

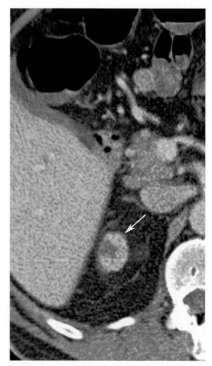

Figure 7.13   B

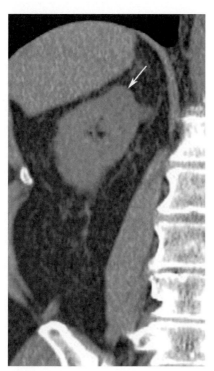

Figure 7.13   C

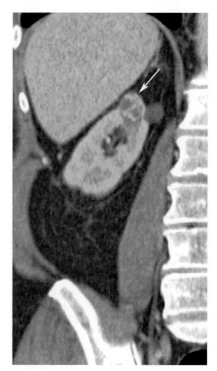

Figure 7.13   D

Findings: Axial unenhanced (A) and nephrographic phase (B) images of the upper pole of the right kidney demonstrate slightly heterogeneously enhancing tissue (arrows) that has the appearance of a cluster of small cysts. On these images alone, a solid renal mass cannot be discerned. Coronal unenhanced (C) and nephrographic phase (D) images reveal a 2.3-cm partially exophytic, heterogeneously enhancing renal mass (arrows) concerning for renal cell carcinoma.

Diagnosis: Renal cell carcinoma, clear cell type

Discussion: This case demonstrates the importance of multiplanar displays in CT urography. When examining the kidney for masses, multiplanar views help detect masses in the poles of the kidney. On axial images, small masses in the poles of the kidney may simulate extensions of the normal kidney, particularly when masses are small and only minimally perturb renal enhancement and contour, as in this case. Images in the coronal or sagittal planes allow for subtle changes in renal enhancement and contour to be seen as separate from the remainder of the kidney. Multiplanar views also depict a renal mass's relationship to surrounding structures and help plan minimally invasive treatment (see Case 7-15).

History: 78-year-old female with abdominal pain.

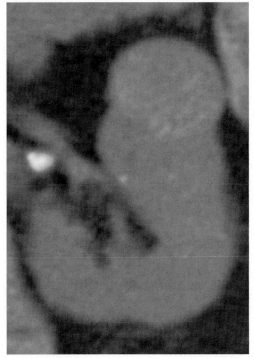

Figure 7.14   A

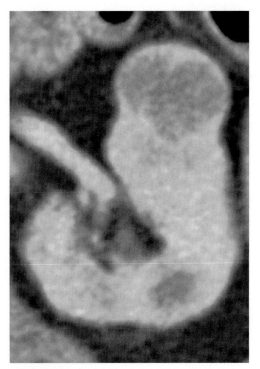

Figure 7.14   B

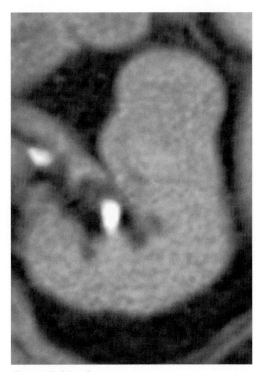

Figure 7.14   C

Findings: Axial unenhanced (A), nephrographic (B), and excretory phase (C) images demonstrate a 2-cm, partially exophytic, hyperdense, enhancing mass in the left kidney. The mass measures 47 HU before contrast material administration, 67 HU on the nephrographic phase image (B), and 75 HU on the excretory phase image (C).

Diagnosis: Renal cell carcinoma, chromophobe type

Discussion: Chromophobe renal cell carcinoma is a subtype of renal cell carcinoma originating from the intercalated cells of the collecting tubules. It is considered an oncocytic renal cell carcinoma and comprises approximately 5% of all renal tumors. Chromophobe renal cell carcinoma has a better prognosis than clear cell renal cell carcinoma for the same stage; the 5-year survival rate is approximately 90%. Chromophobe renal carcinoma, like other oncocytic renal neoplasms, tends to exhibit homogeneous enhancement on CT. At pathology, it shows a homogeneous cut surface without hemorrhage or necrosis and a solid growth pattern. This case is unusual in that the attenuation of the mass is higher during the excretory phase than the nephrographic phase.

History: 57-year-old male with abdominal pain.

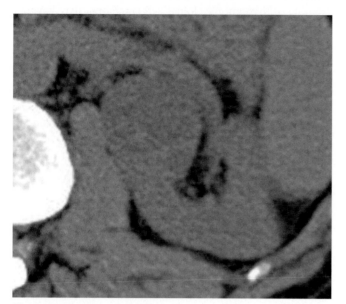

Figure 7.15   A

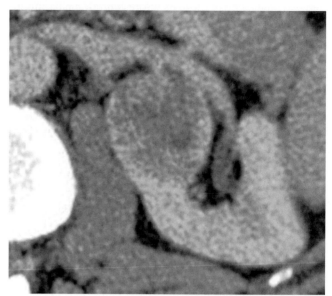

Figure 7.15   B

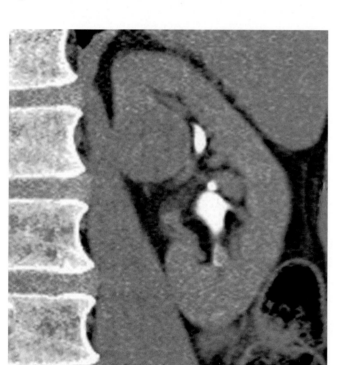

Figure 7.15   C

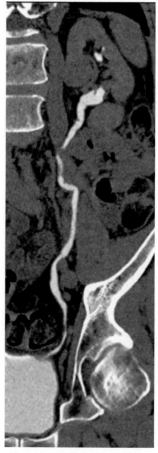

Figure 7.15   D

Findings: Axial unenhanced (A) and enhanced (B) images show an enhancing solid mass in the upper pole of the left kidney. Attenuation of the mass before contrast media administration was 17 HU and after IV contrast media administration was 90 HU. Coronal (C) and curved planar reformatted (D) images during the excretory phase display the relationship of the mass to the renal vein and artery anteriorly (C) and the intrarenal collecting system laterally and inferiorly (D). The apparent filling defects in the ureter (D) are due to ureteral kinking.

Diagnosis: Renal oncocytoma

Discussion: Oncocytoma often appears as a homogeneously enhancing solid mass; however, a characteristic central stellate scar may be present. Another suggestive appearance of oncocytoma is a "spoke wheel" configuration of radiating vessels on angiography. These features should prompt the radiologist to suggest the diagnosis, but they are not pathognomonic. Renal cell carcinoma may have an identical appearance. Oncocytoma is generally considered a benign neoplasm, or one of low malignant potential. Therefore, minimally invasive treatments (e.g., partial nephrectomy and percutaneous tumor ablation) are often employed. Multiplanar and curved planar reformatted images obtained with CT urography display renal masses such that minimally invasive treatments may be planned with knowledge of the mass's relationship to renal vasculature and the intrarenal collecting system and ureter. Rarely, oncocytomas may be multiple and bilateral, a condition referred to as renal oncocytosis.

History: 85-year-old male with intermittent hematuria.

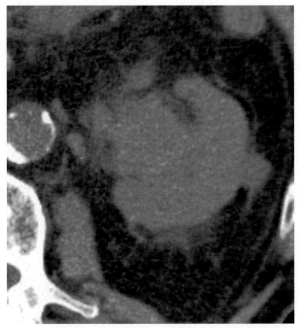

Figure 7.16   A

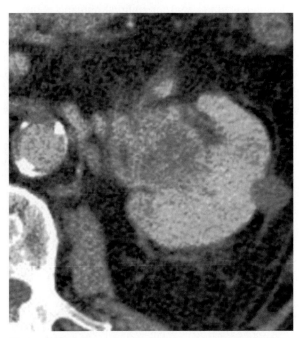

Figure 7.16   B

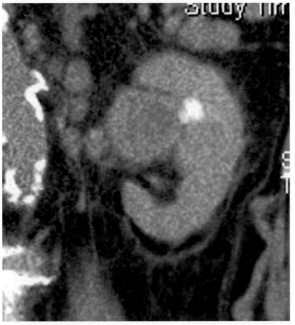

Figure 7.16   C

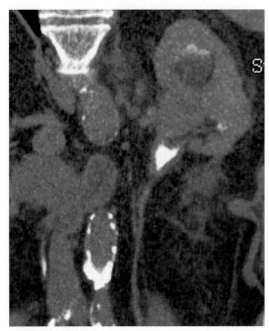

Figure 7.16   D

Findings: Axial unenhanced (A) and nephrographic phase (B) images from a CT urogram demonstrate a 3-cm mass in the left renal sinus with peripheral enhancement. The medial aspect of the mass measures 32 HU on the unenhanced image (A) and 53 HU on the nephrographic phase image (B). Subtle caliectasis is demonstrated on a coronal excretory phase image (C). There is thickening of the proximal left ureter on the curved planar reformatted image (D).

Diagnosis: Transitional cell carcinoma with squamous differentiation

Discussion: The differential diagnosis of an enhancing renal mass includes transitional cell carcinoma (TCC). Masses that are located centrally, either in the renal sinus or adjacent to the renal sinus, should be considered as possibly representing TCC. An accurate preoperative diagnosis is important because renal TCC is treated with nephroureterectomy; renal cell carcinoma is treated with nephrectomy. TCC accounts for 85% to 90% of all uroepithelial tumors. Squamous cell carcinoma accounts for most of the remaining uroepithelial tumors. Occasionally, TCC will display squamous differentiation, as in this case. TCC occurs in urothelial tissue in proportion to surface area. The urinary bladder is the most common location, followed by the renal pelvis and then the ureter. TCC also exhibits a strong tendency toward multiplicity. Approximately 25% of TCCs arising in the renal pelvis or calyx invade the renal parenchyma, as in this case. Lesions in the renal collecting systems can be missed on CT if excretory images are not obtained. This underscores the importance of the excretory phase images obtained during CT urography.

History: 63-year-old male with hypercalcemia.

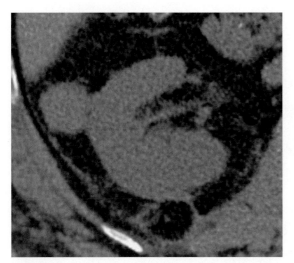

Figure 7.17 A

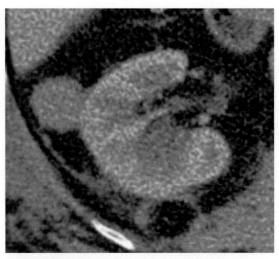

Figure 7.17 B

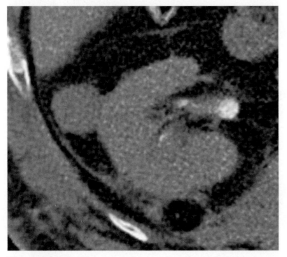

Figure 7.17 C

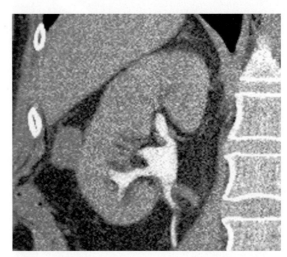

Figure 7.17 D

Findings: Axial unenhanced (A), nephrographic (B), and excretory (C) phase images and coronal excretory phase (D) image from a CT urogram demonstrate a 2-cm homogeneous mass in the interpolar region of the right kidney. The mass enhances homogeneously from 32 HU (A) to 53 HU (B) after contrast media administration. Stranding in the perinephric fat was the result of prior surgery. Coronal image confirms the exophytic nature of the mass and demonstrates no hydronephrosis.

Diagnosis: Renal lymphoma

Discussion: Primary renal lymphoma is rare; however, the kidney is often involved by lymphoma secondarily, either by hematogeneous spread or by direct invasion of adjacent lymphadenopathy. Non-Hodgkin lymphoma is more likely than Hodgkin lymphoma to involve the kidneys. Renal lymphoma can occur with several different patterns. The most common is multifocal, homogeneously enhancing renal parenchymal masses that may have an infiltrative growth pattern. Other patterns of renal involvement of lymphoma include diffuse renal parenchymal infiltration that enlarges one or both kidneys, a solitary renal mass (as in this case), and direct extension into the renal parenchyma or renal sinus from retroperitoneal lymphadenopathy.

History: 61-year-old female with left-sided pain and hematuria.

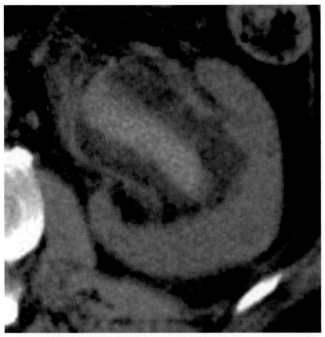

Figure 7.18   A

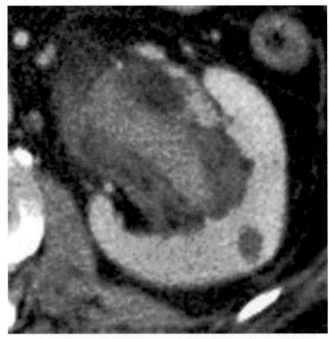

Figure 7.18   B

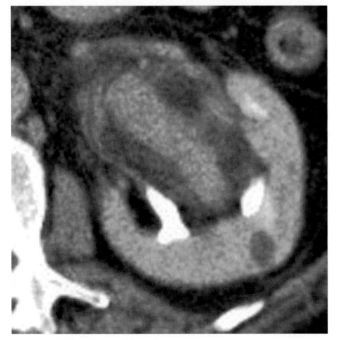

Figure 7.18   C

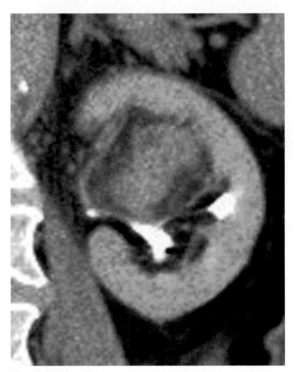

Figure 7.18   D

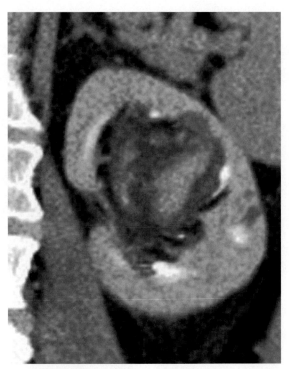

Figure 7.18 E

Findings: Axial unenhanced (A), nephrographic (B) and excretory phase (C) images reveal a 5.6-cm mass in the renal sinus of the upper pole of the left kidney. The mass contains fat attenuation (−48 HU) and a band-shaped region of high attenuation (73 HU) material in its center. Fat stranding in the renal sinus is identified. Coronal images during the excretory phase (D, E) depict the mass as being central but contiguous with and likely arising from renal parenchyma (D).

Diagnosis: Renal angiomyolipoma with intratumoral hemorrhage

Discussion: Angiomyolipoma (AML) is a benign neoplasm containing fat, smooth muscle, and blood vessels. Most renal AMLs (80%) are solitary tumors discovered incidentally in middle-aged women. The remainder are found in patients with tuberous sclerosis. Incidentally diagnosed asymptomatic AMLs do not need treatment. They are diagnosed by identifying fat (CT region of interest measurements of −10 HU or less) within the mass. Other renal masses that contain fat include lipoma, liposarcoma, Wilms' tumor, and, rarely, renal cell carcinoma. However, these are rare. There are several case reports of renal cell carcinomas that contain fat; however, most of them also contain calcifications. Calcifications are rarely found in AMLs. In addition, non-fat-containing tumors may appear to contain fat by engulfing or invading renal sinus or perinephric fat. Thin section images (3–5 mm) should be obtained to minimize the chance of missing fat in AMLs because of partial volume averaging. AMLs have a propensity to bleed because they contain abnormal thin-walled vessels, particularly when they are larger than 4 cm, as in this case. When they do bleed, their appearance may be complex. Coronal images in this case were used to demonstrate the renal origin of the mass and delineate the shape and position of the intratumoral hematoma.

History: 63-year-old female with left flank pain.

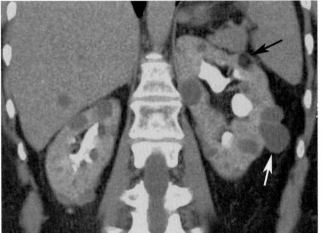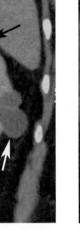

Figure 7.19   A

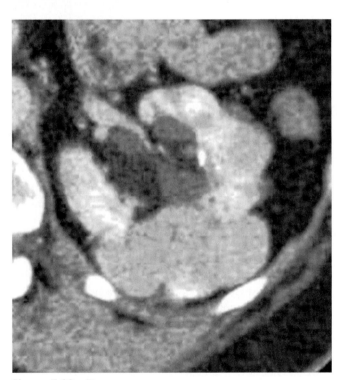

Figure 7.19   B

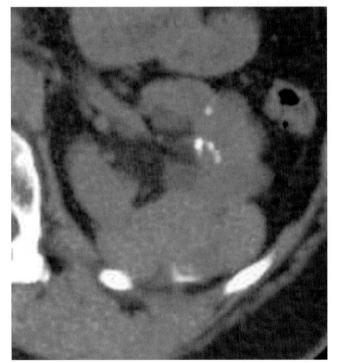

Figure 7.19   C

Figure 7.19   D

Findings: Coronal excretory phase images (A, B) from a CT urogram show multiple cysts in both kidneys [white arrow in (A)], a 1.4-cm fat-containing angiomyolipoma (−63 HU) in the lateral aspect of the upper pole of the left kidney (black arrow) (A), and a 6-cm mass [white arrows in (B)] in the posterolateral aspect of the lower pole of the left kidney. Axial unenhanced image (C) shows that the 6-cm mass is hyperdense (50 HU) and contains subtle,

peripheral calcifications along its posterior aspect. Axial nephrographic phase image (D) shows that the mass enhances to 97 HU.

Diagnosis: Angiomyolipoma with minimal fat

Discussion: Most angiomyolipomas (AMLs) contain a sufficient amount of fat to be detected on imaging studies. The 1.4-cm mass in this case is an example of a fat-containing

AML. If attenuation values more negative than −10 HU can be identified within a noncalcified renal mass, as in the fatty mass illustrated in (A), a diagnosis of AML may be made with confidence. In contrast, some AMLs may contain only a small amount of fat. In these instances, unenhanced CT images may be required to detect the fat because the small amount of fat can be completely obscured once intravenous contrast material has been administered. However, another 4% or 5% of AMLs contain little or no fat and, therefore, fat cannot be identified with imaging. These lesions, also known as AMLs with minimal fat, are composed primarily of smooth muscle and, as a result, are typically hyperdense and enhance homogeneously. The differential diagnosis for hyperdense,

homogeneously enhancing renal masses also includes malignant lesions such as renal cell carcinoma (particularly papillary subtype), metastases, and benign lesions such as oncocytoma, metanephric adenoma, and leiomyoma. Since the differential diagnosis includes both benign and malignant lesions, percutaneous biopsy could be considered before treatment. The 6-cm mass in the lower pole in this case was also proven to be an AML with minimal fat by percutaneous biopsy. The presence of multiple AMLs and cysts should raise the possibility of tuberous sclerosis (see Case 7-20) in this patient. However, there was no family history or other signs of tuberous sclerosis.

History: 23-year-old female with bilateral flank pain.

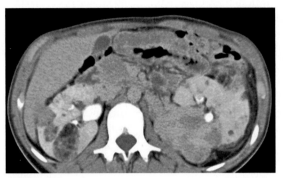

Figure 7.20 A

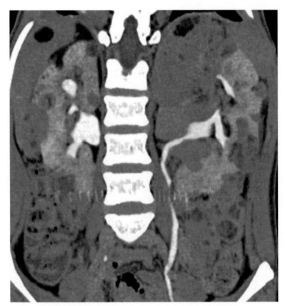

Figure 7.20 B

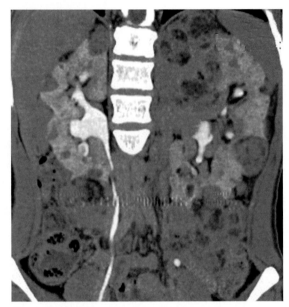

Figure 7.20 C

Findings: Axial (A) image and curved planar reformatted images (B, C) during the excretory phase from a CT urogram demonstrate markedly enlarged kidneys with multiple masses containing areas of fat attenuation (<−10 HU) diagnostic of multiple angiomyolipomas (AMLs). Some of the masses contain little or no fat. Multiple cystic masses are also present. Curved planar reformatted images (B, C) during the excretory phase demonstrate that the collecting systems are secondarily compressed and distorted by the multiple masses. Curved planar reformations also demonstrate innumerable masses extending into the perinephric spaces. An AML is also incidentally seen in the liver.

Diagnosis: Tuberous sclerosis

Discussion: Innumerable fat-containing renal masses are diagnostic of tuberous sclerosis, an autosomal dominant hereditary disorder characterized by the triad of facial adenoma sebaceum, periventricular hamartomas in the brain, and mental retardation. Other nonrenal manifestations of tuberous sclerosis include pulmonary lymphangioleiomyomatosis, cardiac rhabdomyomas, cutaneous shagreen patches, and, as in this case, hepatic AMLs. Multiple renal AMLs are the most common and characteristic manifestation of tuberous sclerosis in the genitourinary system. Eighty percent of patients with tuberous sclerosis develop renal AMLs. When larger than 4 cm in diameter, AMLs may bleed and require angiographic embolization or nephrectomy. The AMLs are typically composed of mostly fat; however, in this case, some of them contain little or no fat. CT urography protocols that include thin section images are often helpful in detecting small amounts of fat.

Multiple renal cysts may occur also in patients with tuberous sclerosis and rarely may predominate.

History: 58-year-old male on dialysis for end-stage renal disease with hematuria.

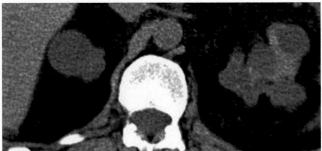

Figure 7.21   A

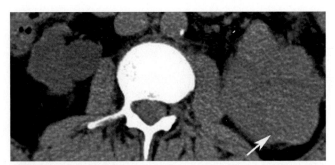

Figure 7.21   B

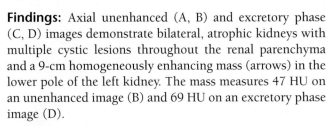

Figure 7.21   C

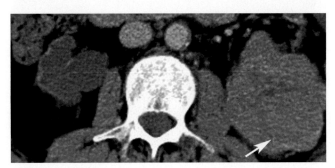

Figure 7.21   D

Findings: Axial unenhanced (A, B) and excretory phase (C, D) images demonstrate bilateral, atrophic kidneys with multiple cystic lesions throughout the renal parenchyma and a 9-cm homogeneously enhancing mass (arrows) in the lower pole of the left kidney. The mass measures 47 HU on an unenhanced image (B) and 69 HU on an excretory phase image (D).

Diagnosis: Acquired cystic kidney disease with renal cell carcinoma

Discussion: Acquired cystic kidney disease is a cystic nephropathy that is the result of the development of multiple cysts primarily in the native kidneys of patients with end-stage renal disease on long-term hemodialysis. However, it also occurs in patients with chronic renal failure not receiving dialysis as well as in the native kidneys of renal transplant recipients with good graft function. Approximately 90% of patients on dialysis for 5 years develop acquired cystic kidney disease. Acquired cystic kidney disease affects men more than women, and blacks are affected nearly twice as often as whites. Affected kidneys are usually small and atrophic, as in this case. The cysts are predominantly cortical, usually bilateral, and number at least four in each kidney. The incidence of the disease, and both the number and the size of cysts, increases in proportion to the duration of dialysis. Most patients are asymptomatic, but some may present with hematuria, flank pain, or a palpable renal mass. Persistent or severe hemorrhage may necessitate nephrectomy or renal embolization. It has also been reported that the incidence of renal cell carcinoma in patients on dialysis is 57 to 134 times higher than in the general population. Most of these are low-grade neoplasms. Invasive renal cell carcinoma is only five times more common in patients with acquired cystic kidney disease than in the general population. Once cysts are observed sonographically, further evaluation with contrast-enhanced CT may be indicated to exclude carcinoma.

History: 69-year-old male with vague abdominal pain.

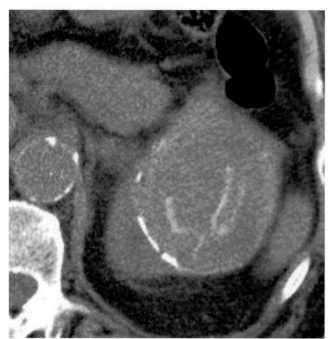

Figure 7.22   A

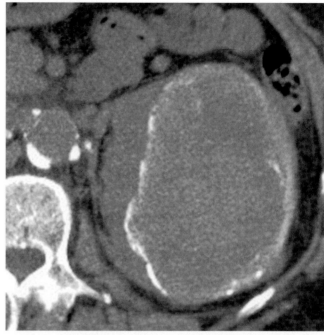

Figure 7.22   B

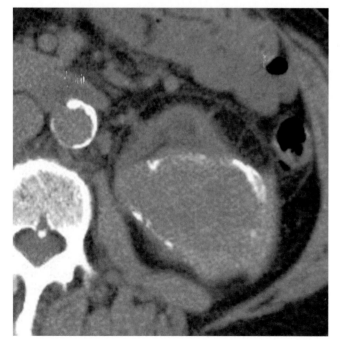

Figure 7.22   C

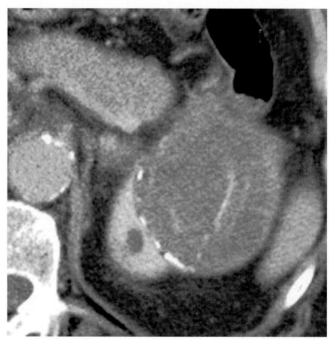

Figure 7.22   D

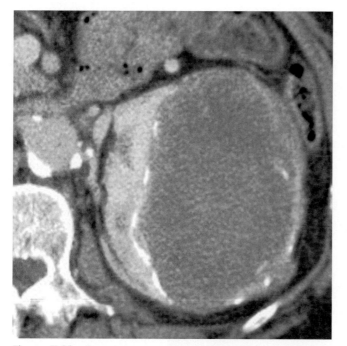

Figure 7.22   E

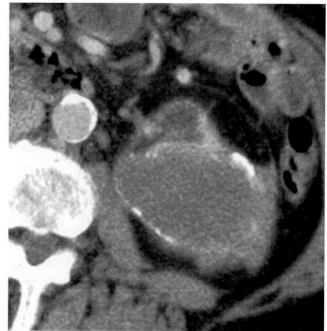

Figure 7.22   F

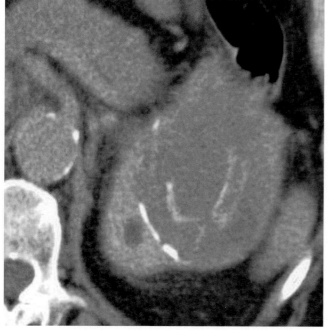

Figure 7.22   G

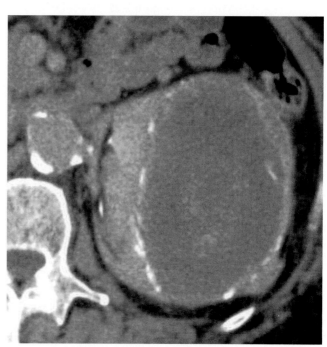

Figure 7.22   H

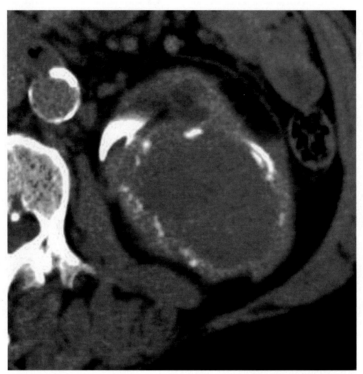

Figure 7.22   I

Findings: Axial unenhanced (A–C), nephrographic phase (D–F), and excretory phase (G–I) images reveal a 10-cm mass in the left kidney. On the unenhanced images, the mass is heterogeneously hyperdense, with an attenuation of 46 HU, and calcified both centrally and peripherally. There are no portions of the mass that enhance. Minimal perinephric stranding is present.

Diagnosis: Renal hematoma

Discussion: Renal hematomas can mimic renal neoplasms, particularly when they are chronic. The inciting traumatic event is often long forgotten and the inflammatory signs of perinephric stranding that usually accompany acute hematomas have largely resolved. As a result, a chronic hematoma may mimic a solid neoplasm by consisting of high-attenuation (>20 HU) tissue and calcifications. However, renal hematomas do not enhance. Since renal cell cancer almost always enhances, hematoma should be considered when a peripherally calcified, nonenhancing renal mass is encountered. Rarely, enhancement will not be found in renal cancers, particularly the papillary subtype. Therefore, this mass was thought to possibly represent a large, nonenhancing renal cell carcinoma, and it was resected.

History: 77-year-old male with an incidental finding.

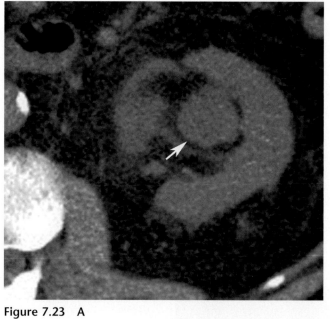

Figure 7.23 A

Figure 7.23 B

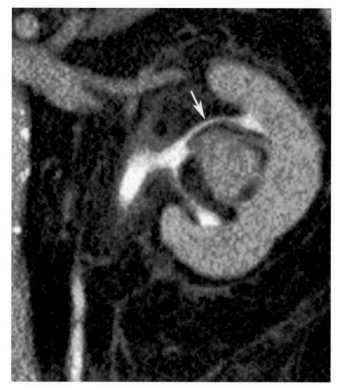

Figure 7.23 C

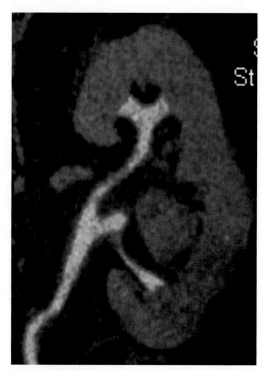

Figure 7.23 D

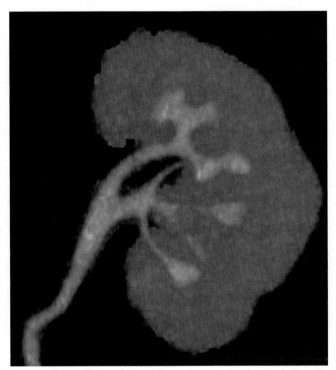

Figure 7.23 E

Findings: Axial unenhanced (A) and nephrographic (B) images from a CT urogram demonstrate a 2.7-cm mass (arrows) positioned in the renal sinus of the left kidney. Portions of the mass measure 19 HU before and 92 HU after contrast material administration. Coronal (C), curved planar reformatted (D), and maximum intensity projection (E) images, all obtained during the excretory phase, demonstrate that the mass is separate from renal parenchyma and displaces an infundibulum superiorly (arrow). These images suggest that the mass arises from the renal sinus and not from the kidney or the collecting system. There is stranding in the periureteral fat.

Diagnosis: Vascular malformation, partially thrombosed, renal sinus

Discussion: Not all enhancing renal masses are solid neoplasms. Inflammatory processes and vascular abnormalities may also enhance and, therefore, mimic neoplasms. CT urography was valuable in this case by defining the mass anatomically as a renal sinus lesion and not a renal parenchymal mass, thus providing an important clue to the diagnosis. The renal sinus consists of perirenal fat, blood vessels, lymphatics, and the renal collecting system. By knowing what resides in the renal sinus, an appropriate differential diagnosis may be constructed. An unusual soft tissue neoplasm, such as an undifferentiated liposarcoma, could be considered, but these are usually larger at presentation. Renal vascular malformations can be classified as congenital, acquired, or spontaneous. Seventy-five percent of arteriovenous communications are acquired. The remainder are congenital. Nearly all acquired lesions are related to natural or iatrogenic penetrating trauma, including nephrectomy and needle biopsy. Less commonly, an eroding neoplasm causes a spontaneous arteriovenous fistula. Spontaneous arteriovenous fistulae usually complicate primary renal artery disease, such as renal artery dissection or renal artery aneurysm rupture. Patients may present with hematuria or hypertension. Large vascular malformations may cause shunts that produce a bruit over the involved kidney and high-flow congestive heart failure. Arteriography provides the definitive diagnosis. Both acquired and spontaneous vascular malformations typically consist of a single feeding artery to a single draining vein. Congenital arteriovenous malformations, referred to as cirsoid aneurysms because of the tangle of small vessels that make up the lesions, demonstrate varixlike communications between the artery and vein. CT may demonstrate a mass effect or impression on the renal collecting system, as in this case, as well as intense enhancement of the involved portion of the kidney. Transcatheter embolization is the treatment of choice in patients with persistent and symptomatic spontaneous or acquired benign arteriovenous malformations.

CASE 7-24

History: 32-year-old female with left lower quadrant pain and an incidental finding.

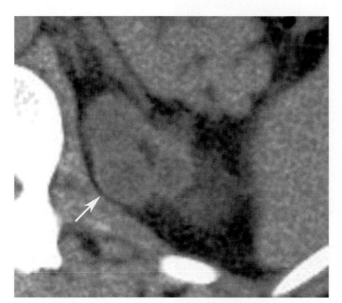

Figure 7.24   A

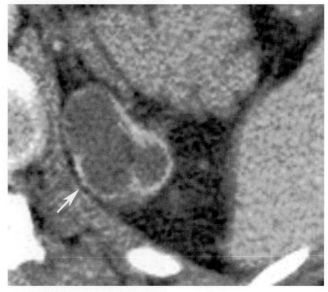

Figure 7.24   B

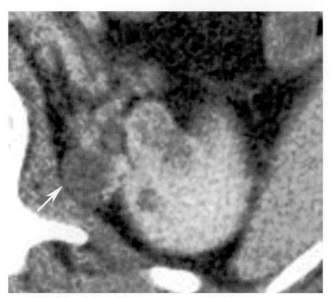

Figure 7.24   C

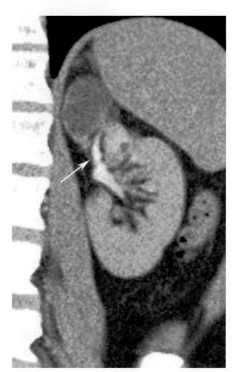

Figure 7.24   D

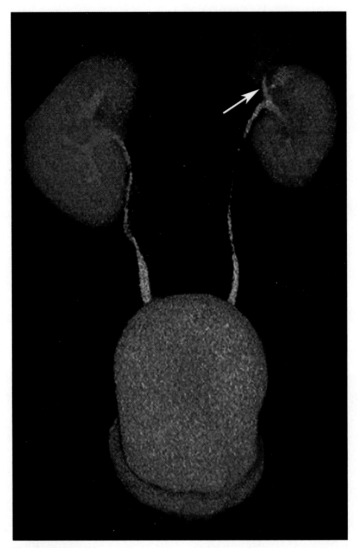

Figure 7.24   E

Findings: Axial unenhanced (A) and nephrographic phase images (B, C) from a CT urogram demonstrate a 4-cm cystic masslike lesion (arrows) in the upper pole of the left kidney. The lesion has the appearance of a hydronephrotic upper pole (dilated calices surrounding sinus fat). Coronal (D) and volume-rendered (E) images during the excretory phase demonstrate an upper pole infundibulum (arrows). The upper pole of the kidney is smaller than the normal-appearing, lower portion of the kidney.

Diagnosis: Segmental multicystic dysplasia

Discussion: This mass was interpreted as a renal tumor using an abdominal CT scan obtained at an outside hospital. The patient was referred to a urologist at our institution for resection. CT urography was able to show that the masslike structure was a dysplastic upper pole, as evidenced by upper pole hydronephrosis and an opacified upper pole infundibulum and by renal parenchymal tissue

loss. Multicystic dysplastic kidney is a developmental abnormality characterized by multiple noncommunicating cysts of variable size with no intervening normal renal parenchyma, resulting from early in utero urinary tract obstruction. It is the most common cause of an abdominal mass in the newborn period and the most common cystic malformation of the kidney in infancy. It occurs sporadically and is not genetic. When multicystic dysplastic kidney is confined to a portion of the kidney, the abnormality is called segmental multicystic dysplasia. Segmental multicystic dysplasia is usually associated with ureteral duplication and obstruction of the upper pole moiety of a duplicated collecting system by either intrinsic narrowing or a ureterocele. Although a duplicated ureter was not identified in this case, it is conceivable that the duplicated ureter was threadlike and invisible.

SUGGESTED READINGS

1. Blumethal I. Vesicoureteric reflux and urinary tract infection in children. *Postgrad Med J.* 2006;82:31–35.

2. Bosniak MA. The small (less than or equal to 3.0 cm) renal parenchymal tumor: detection, diagnosis, and controversies. *Radiology.* 1991;179:307–317.

3. Bosniak MA. Problems in the radiologic diagnosis of renal parenchymal tumors. *Urol Clin North Am.* 1993;20:217–230.

4. Browne RFJ, Meehan CP, Colville J, et al. Transitional cell carcinoma of the upper urinary tract: spectrum of findings. *Radiographics.* 2005;25:1609–1627.

5. Casper KA, Donnelly LF, Chen B, et al. Tuberous sclerosis complex: renal imaging findings. *Radiology.* 2002;225:451–456.

6. Crotty KL, Orihuela E, Warren MM. Recent advances in the diagnosis and treatment of renal arteriovascular malformations and fistulas. *J Urol.* 1993;150:1355–1359.

7. Davidson AJ, Hayes WS, Hartman DS, et al. Renal oncocytoma and carcinoma: failure of differentiation with CT. *Radiology.* 1993;186: 693–696.

8. Dyer RB, Chen MY, Zagoria RJ. Classic signs in uroradiology. *Radiographics.* 2004;24:S247–S280.

9. Fallon B, Williams RD. Renal cancer associated with acquired cystic disease of the kidney and chronic renal failure. *Semin Urol.* 1989;7:228–236.

10. Gabow PA. Autosomal dominant polycystic kidney disease: more than a renal disease. *Am J Kidney Dis.* 1990;16:403–413.

11. Gupta S, Seith A, Sud K, et al. CT in the evaluation of complicated autosomal dominant polycystic kidney disease. *Acta Radiol.* 2000;41: 280–284.

12. Israel GM, Bosniak MA. Follow-up CT of moderately complex cystic lesions of the kidney: Bosniak category IIF. *Am J Roentgenol.* 2003;181:627–633.

13. Jeon A, Cramer BC, Walsh E, et al. A spectrum of segmental multicystic renal dysplasia. *Pediatr Radiol.* 1999;29:309–315.

14. Jinzaki M, McTavish JD, Zou KH, et al. Evaluation of small (≤3 cm) renal masses with MDCT: benefits of thin overlapping reconstructions. *Am J Roentgenol.* 2004;183:223–228.

15. Jinzaki M, Tanimoto A, Narimatsu Y, et al. Angiomyolipoma: imaging findings in lesions with minimal fat. *Radiology.* 1997;205:497–502.

16. Kawashima A, Sandler CM, Corl FM, et al. Imaging of renal trauma: a comprehensive review. *Radiographics.* 2001;21:557–574.

17. Kim JK, Kim TK, Ahn HJ, et al. Differentiation of subtypes of renal cell carcinoma on helical CT scans. *Am J Roentgenol.* 2002;178: 1499–1506.

18. Macari M, Bosniak MA. Delayed CT to evaluate renal masses incidentally discovered at contrast-enhanced CT: demonstration of vascularity with deenhancement. *Radiology.* 1999;213:674–680.

19. Quinn MJ, Hartman DS, Friedman AC, et al. Renal oncocytoma: new observations. *Radiology.* 1984;153:49–53.

20. Silverman SG, Gan YU, Mortele KJ, et al. Renal masses in the adult patient: the role of percutaneous biopsy. *Radiology.* 2006;240:6–22.

21. Urban BA, Fishman EK. Renal lymphoma: CT patterns with emphasis on helical CT. *Radiographics.* 2000;20:197–212.

CHAPTER EIGHT

INTRARENAL COLLECTING SYSTEM

TERRI J. VRTISKA, MD

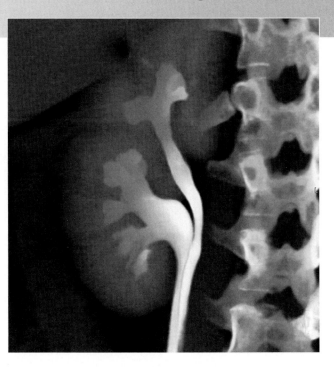

History: 69-year-old female with microscopic hematuria and recurrent stone disease.

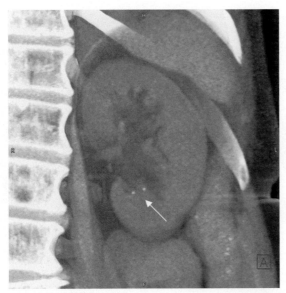

Figure 8.1 A

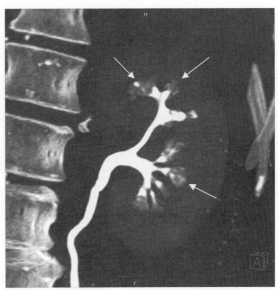

Figure 8.1 B

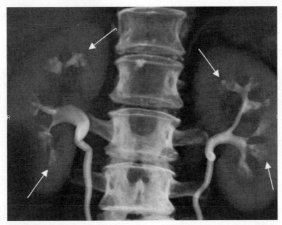

Figure 8.1 C

Findings: Unenhanced volume rendered coronal image of the left kidney (A) demonstrates two small calculi in the lower pole of the left kidney (arrow). Enhanced maximum intensity projection image of the left kidney obtained during the excretory phase (B) and enhanced volume rendered image of both kidneys also obtained during the excretory phase (C) demonstrate multiple brushlike and round collections of contrast material throughout the papillae of both kidneys (arrows).

Diagnosis: Medullary sponge kidney

Discussion: Renal tubular ectasia is diagnosed by identifying linear collections of contrast material in the collecting ducts appearing as linear, paint brush-like striations (see Cases 4-10 and 11-2). The discrete linear collections (that resemble a paint brush) should not be confused with the indistinct normal papillary "blush" (see Case 4-2). Relative to CT in the past, the improved spatial resolution of multidetector CT allows for both the diagnosis and the depiction of the extent of this abnormality of the upper urinary tract collecting system.

One or more papillae may be affected. The findings are bilateral in 60% to 80% of cases. The isolated finding of linear collections is termed benign renal tubular ectasia. When the collections are cystic and associated with urolithiasis or medullary nephrocalcinosis, as in this case, the term medullary sponge kidney can be applied. Clinical presentation includes infection, symptomatic stone disease, and/or hematuria.

History: 19-year-old female status post bilateral ureteral reimplantation for reflux nephropathy.

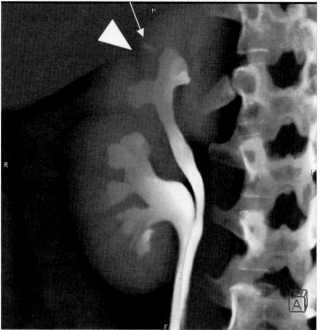

Figure 8.2   A

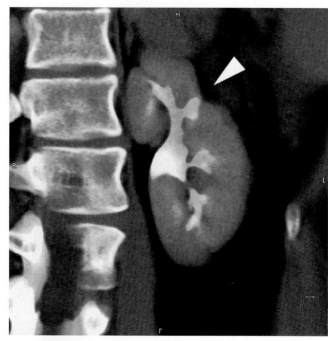

Figure 8.2   B

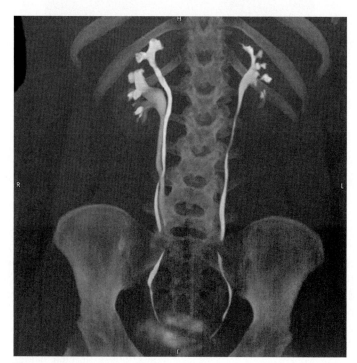

Figure 8.2   C

Findings: Coronal volume rendered combined nephrographic/excretory phase images of the right (A) and left (B) kidneys and the entire urinary tract (C) from a CT urogram using the split bolus technique demonstrate duplication of the right intrarenal collecting system and ureter. There are bilateral parenchymal scars, particularly in the upper poles of both kidneys (arrowheads). In the right upper pole, there is a small, linear-shaped collection (arrow) of contrast material in the papilla adjacent to a scar. There is also mild caliectasis bilaterally.

Diagnosis: Reflux nephropathy (chronic pyelonephritis)

Discussion: Historically, reflux nephropathy has been referred to as chronic pyelonephritis (see Cases 6-10 and 7-1) and is associated with vesicoureteric reflux (VUR).

However, reflux nephropathy is the preferred term because the changes seen in this condition almost always result from VUR during childhood. Although VUR often disappears during adulthood, the resulting mild caliectasis and renal parenchymal scars persist. Renal parenchymal scarring that results from reflux nephropathy can be differentiated from scarring due to renal infarcts. Ischemic infarcts are limited to the cortex and do not affect the underlying calyces, whereas reflux nephropathy scars involve the full thickness of the renal parenchyma and are associated with caliectasis. Reflux nephropathy can lead to progressive renal failure in adults. Approximately 10% to 20% of patients requiring dialysis or renal transplantation are due to progressive renal parenchymal loss from reflux nephropathy.

History: 39-year-old female with microscopic hematuria, flank pain, and a right-sided ureterocele on cystoscopy.

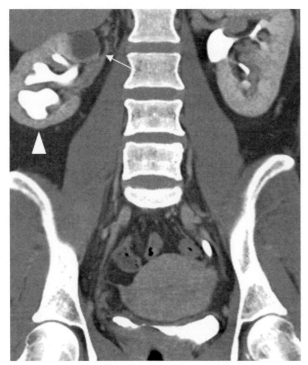

Figure 8.3   A

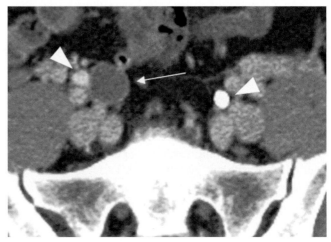

Figure 8.3   B

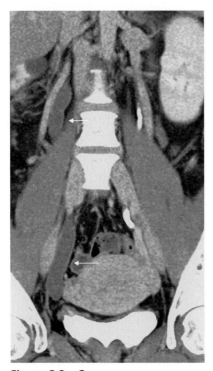

Figure 8.3   C

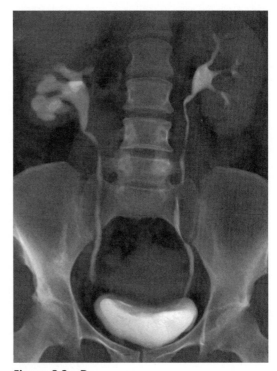

Figure 8.3   D

Findings: Coronal thick slab maximum intensity projection images (A, C), axial image (B), and volume rendered image (D) obtained during the excretory phase of a CT urogram performed using split bolus technique demonstrate a nonopacified cystic lesion in the upper pole of the right kidney [arrow in (A)] as well as moderate dilatation and parenchymal scarring of the lower pole of the right kidney [arrowhead in (A)]. Opacified ureteral segments are noted on the axial CT image [arrowheads in (B)]. An unopacified tubular structure, consistent with a dilated ureter of an obstructed right upper pole moiety, is best demonstrated on the thick coronal maximum intensity projection series [arrows in (C)], a segment of which is also seen on the axial image [arrow in (B)]. The volume rendered image (D) demonstrates only the opacified intrarenal collecting systems and ureters bilaterally. The unopacified right upper pole renal collecting system can only be suspected by its impression upon the lower pole renal collecting system. These findings combined with a ureterocele noted at cystoscopy are consistent with an obstructed right upper pole moiety of a duplicated intrarenal collecting system as well as with vesicoureteral reflux and scarring in the lower pole moiety.

Diagnosis: Ureteral duplication with upper pole moiety obstruction and lower pole moiety reflux

Discussion: The findings of a duplicated system, a dilated upper pole moiety ureter, lower pole atrophy, and a ureterocele detected at cystoscopy are consistent with an obstructed upper pole moiety of a duplicated intrarenal collecting system as well as with vesicoureteral reflux and scarring of the lower moiety of the right kidney. In this case, chronic obstruction led to parenchymal loss and cystic change in the right renal parenchyma. However, in other cases, the upper pole moiety may be markedly hydronephrotic; the resultant extensive downward displacement of the lower pole moiety causes the "drooping lily" sign. Duplication of the intrarenal collecting system and ureter is a common, often asymptomatic congenital anomaly. Some form of collecting system duplication anomaly is found in 15% of patients. A consistent relationship of the duplicated ureters' insertions into the bladder occurs in 85% of patients: The upper pole moiety ureter inserts in a position inferior and medial to the lower pole moiety ureter. This anatomic relationship is known as the Weigert–Meyer rule. The upper pole moiety ureteral insertion site in the bladder is ectopic (i.e., located in an anomalous position either in or outside the bladder). The ectopic ureter is also often associated with a ureterocele.

History: 28-year-old male with history of stone disease.

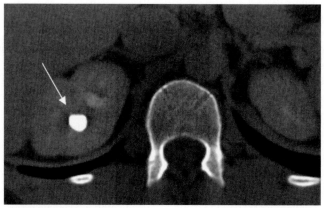

Figure 8.4 A

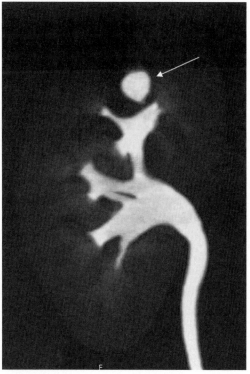

Figure 8.4 B

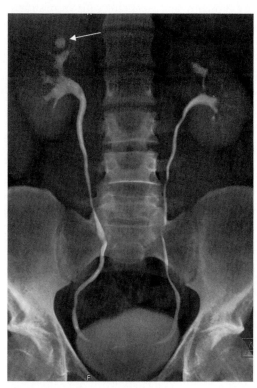

Figure 8.4 C

Findings: Axial image of the right kidney (A), coronal maximal intensity projection image of the right kidney (B), and volume rendered image of both kidneys (C) obtained during the excretory phase of a CT urogram demonstrate a well-circumscribed contrast material-filled structure (arrows) arising from an upper pole calyx of the right kidney. Images (B) and (C) best demonstrate the communication of the structure with the normal right intrarenal collecting system via a narrow isthmus from an upper pole fornix.

Diagnosis: Congenital calyceal diverticulum

Discussion: A congenital calyceal diverticulum is a urothelial-lined outpouching of the urinary collecting system that is connected to a peripheral calyx via a thin necklike infundibulum most commonly in the upper or lower pole of the kidney (see Case 7-5). Approximately one-third of diverticula are complicated by stone disease (see Case 4-13). Additional complications include infection and abscess formation, which may necessitate treatment such as stone extraction or ablation.

On standard CT images obtained prior to excretion of contrast media into the renal collecting systems, these appear as water attenuation masses and are likely to be confused with cystic renal masses or abscesses. However, congenital calyceal diverticula generally can be differentiated from these lesions because they opacify with contrast material on the excretory phase images obtained during CT urography due to their communication with the renal collecting system. Renal cysts and abscesses rarely communicate with the intrarenal collecting system (see Case 6-4).

Coronal images acquired with CT urography are helpful for depicting the anatomic relationship of the diverticulum with the rest of the intrarenal collecting system, prior to percutaneous interventional treatment or surgery.

History: 57-year-old male with history of gross hematuria. Medications include nonsteroidal anti-inflammatory drugs (NSAIDs), aspirin, and acetaminophen.

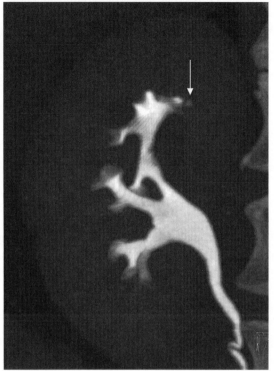

Figure 8.5   A

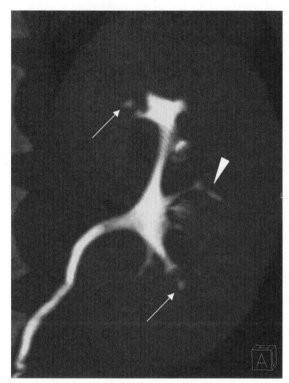

Figure 8.5   B

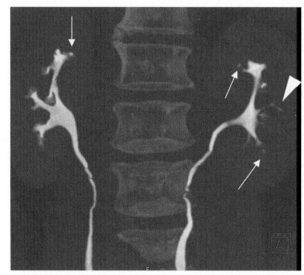

Figure 8.5   C

Findings: Coronal maximum intensity projection images obtained during the excretory phase of a CT urogram including localized views of the right kidney (A), the left kidney (B), and both kidneys (C) demonstrate a small extracalyceal contrast material-containing collection involving the upper pole of the right kidney [arrows over right kidney in (A) and (C)] and several small extracalyceal contrast material-containing collections involving the upper and lower pole of the left kidney [arrows over left kidney in (B) and (C)] as well as an eccentric linear collection extending into the lateral midportion of the left kidney [arrowheads in (B) and (C)].

Diagnosis: Papillary necrosis

Discussion: Papillary necrosis may present in patients with flank pain, hematuria, or decreased renal function. It can develop as a result of vascular compromise, infection, or obstruction of the sensitive renal papillae (see Case 6-9).

Some of the traditional causes of papillary necrosis are no longer a concern clinically (e.g., phenacetin). However, papillary necrosis is associated with the ingestion of several currently used medications (e.g., NSAIDs) as well as common underlying medical conditions (diabetes, urinary tract infection, sickle cell anemia, and sickle cell trait). Changes of papillary necrosis demonstrated by CT urography are due to tracking of excreted contrast material into central or eccentric papillary cavities that communicate with calyces. Additional findings include calyceal blunting and renal parenchymal scarring. The "lobster-claw" sign of papillary necrosis is due to complete sloughing of the central papilla with distortion of a residual "claw-shaped" calyx. Rare findings include filling defects within the collecting system due to the total amputation and sloughing of papillae.

History: 83-year-old male with history of diabetes, stone disease, hematuria, and flank pain.

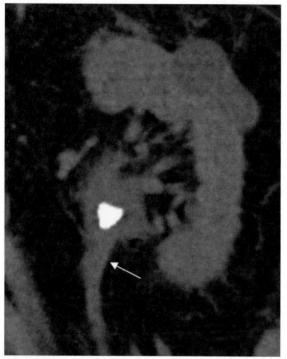

Figure 8.6   A

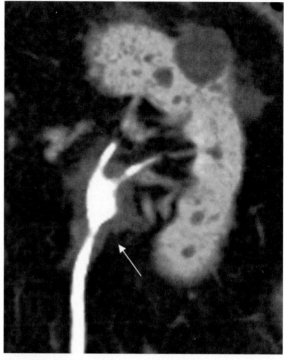

Figure 8.6   B

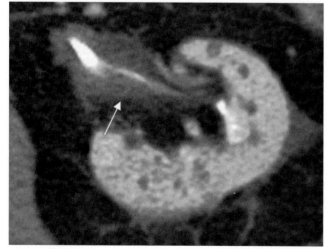

Figure 8.6   C

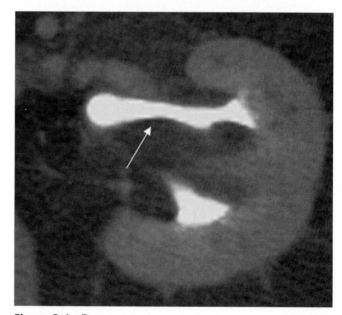

Figure 8.6   D

Findings: Coronal maximum intensity projection images without IV contrast material (A) and with excreted contrast material (B) are obtained from a CT urogram using the split bolus technique. These images, along with an axial combined nephrographic/excretory phase image of the mid left kidney (C), show moderate circumferential thickening of the left renal pelvis wall (arrows). After treatment, resolution of the urothelial wall thickening occurred, as confirmed by an excretory phase image from a CT urogram obtained 6 months later [(D), arrow].

Diagnosis: Pyelitis

Discussion: Pyelitis is a benign inflammatory condition of the renal pelvis commonly due to urinary calculi or infection (see Case 5-2). The urothelium of the entire renal pelvis becomes inflamed, and the inflammation may extend into the renal parenchyma with resultant pyelonephritis. Associated urinary tract obstruction can result in distention of the intrarenal collecting system with development of pyonephrosis. The most important differential diagnosis is transitional cell carcinoma (TCC), and cystoscopy/ureteroscopy may be necessary to exclude neoplasm. Follow-up CT urography can be obtained to document stability or resolution of the findings after the inflammation subsides.

History: 77-year-old male with retroperitoneal sarcoma.

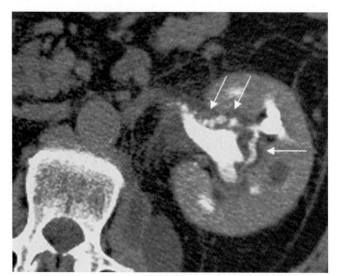

Figure 8.7   A

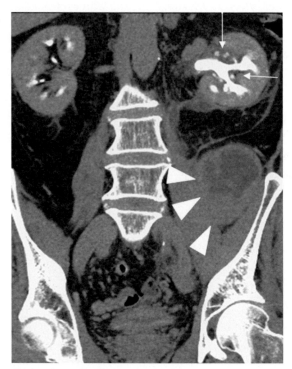

Figure 8.7   B

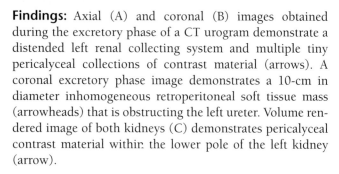

Figure 8.7   C

Findings: Axial (A) and coronal (B) images obtained during the excretory phase of a CT urogram demonstrate a distended left renal collecting system and multiple tiny pericalyceal collections of contrast material (arrows). A coronal excretory phase image demonstrates a 10-cm in diameter inhomogeneous retroperitoneal soft tissue mass (arrowheads) that is obstructing the left ureter. Volume rendered image of both kidneys (C) demonstrates pericalyceal contrast material within the lower pole of the left kidney (arrow).

Diagnosis: Forniceal rupture with contrast material extravasation (pyelosinus backflow) due to ureteral obstruction by leiomyosarcoma

Discussion: Obstruction of normal urine flow results in increased pressure within the collecting system and occasionally may result in decompression (backflow) into adjacent structures, especially when the increased pressure occurs suddenly (as in patients who present acutely with ureterolithiasis or during retrograde pyelography) (see Case

5-5). In some instances, as in this case, such decompression can occur in patients with chronic obstruction. Backflow can be diagnosed on CT urography when excreted contrast material is observed to have extravasated outside of the renal collecting system (see Case 9-18).

Five types of backflow have been described: pyelotubular backflow into the collecting ducts, pyelointerstitial backflow into the adjacent interstitium, pyelosinus backflow into the adjacent renal sinus, pyelovenous backflow into an adjacent renal vein, and pyelolymphatic backflow into the lymphatic system. Pyelolymphatic and pyelosinus backflow have been observed during both intravenous urography and CT urography. Pyelovenous backflow has also been demonstrated on CT urography when ureteral obstruction is associated with obstruction of the renal vein or the inferior vena cava. When backflow of any type occurs, the process is usually self-limited. Any extravasated urine and contrast material is almost always resorbed rapidly without any adverse sequelae. However, if the extravasated urine is infected, retroperitoneal abscesses can develop.

History: 72-year-old male with history of hematuria and stone disease.

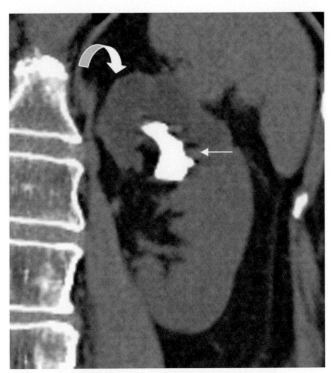

Figure 8.8   A

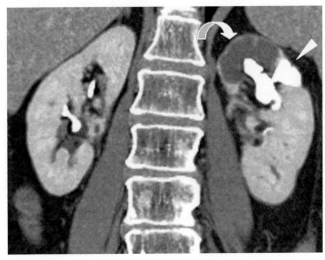

Figure 8.8   C

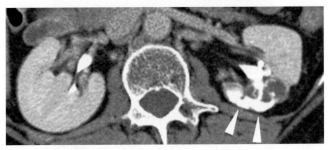

Figure 8.8   B

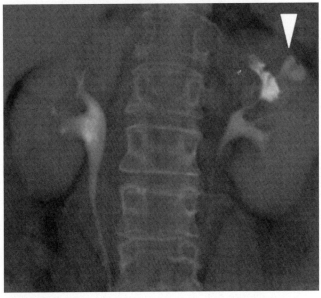

Figure 8.8   D

Findings: Unenhanced coronal image (A) demonstrates a branched calculus in the upper pole of the left kidney (arrow) with a peripheral low-attenuation area in the adjacent renal parenchyma (curved arrow). Axial CT (B), coronal CT (C), and volume-rendered (D) images obtained in a combined nephrographic/excretory phase of a CT urogram performed with the split bolus technique demonstrate dilatation of the left upper pole calyces and marked thinning of the renal parenchyma in the left upper pole (arrowheads). The low-attenuation area (curved arrow), which has a lobulated shape, is contiguous with the branched calculus.

Diagnosis: Branched calculus with upper pole hydrocalyx

Discussion: Focal hydronephrosis (hydrocalyx and hydrocalycosis) results from obstruction of a draining renal segment due to inflammatory changes, stone disease, or tumor. Hydrocalyx can be suspected on unenhanced images when there are low-attenuation changes in the affected renal segment. Opacification of the dilated calyces often requires markedly delayed excretory phase images. In this case, the lobulated contour of the low-attenuation left upper pole structures and their contiguity with the branched calculus suggests that they represent markedly dilated obstructed calyces.

History: 86-year-old female with history of transitional cell carcinoma of the bladder.

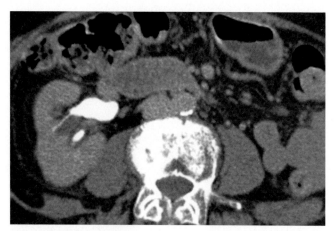

Figure 8.9   A

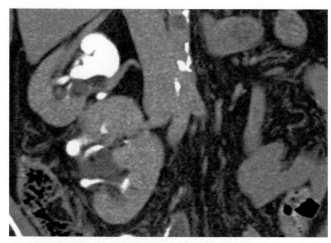

Figure 8.9   B

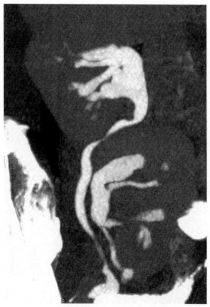

Figure 8.9   C

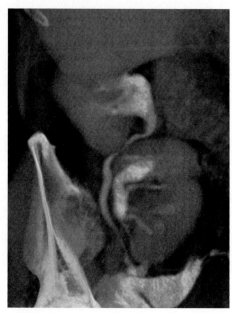

Figure 8.9   D

Findings: Axial excretory phase image (A) demonstrates absence of the left kidney in the left renal fossa. Coronal (B), maximum intensity projection (C), and volume-rendered (D) images obtained during the excretory phase of CT urography demonstrate both kidneys on the right side of the abdomen.

Diagnosis: Crossfused renal ectopia

Discussion: Developmental anomalies of the kidneys include renal ectopia such as crossfused renal ectopia (see Case 4-16). Most commonly, the left kidney is aberrant and fused to the right kidney. There are invariably aberrant arteries; however, typically, the ureter draining the crossed kidney inserts on the normal contralateral side of the bladder. CT urography, especially with use of three-dimensional and multiplanar reformatted images, is helpful for determining the anatomic relationships of the arteries, veins, intrarenal collecting systems, and ureters. Complications of crossfused renal ectopia include infection and stone disease.

CASE 8-10

History: 71-year-old male with history of hematuria.

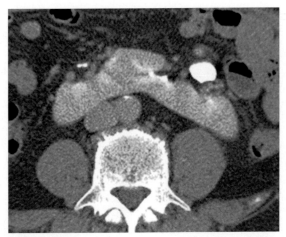

Figure 8.10   A

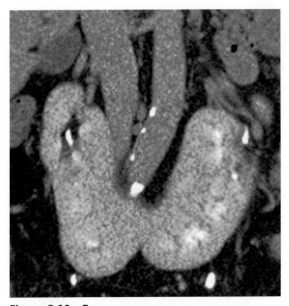

Figure 8.10   B

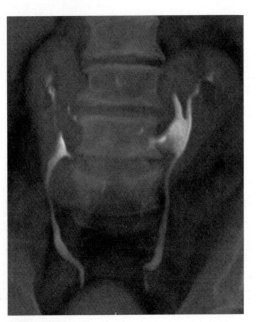

Figure 8.10   C

Findings: An axial image (A), a thick slab coronal maximum intensity projection image (B), and a volume-rendered image of both kidneys (C) obtained during the combined nephrographic/pyelographic phase of a CT urogram performed using the split bolus technique demonstrate midline fusion of the kidneys.

Diagnosis: Renal fusion anomaly (horseshoe kidney)

Discussion: Fusion anomalies of the kidneys, such as horseshoe kidney, result from abnormalities that occur early in embryological development (see Case 4-9). With horseshoe kidneys, the lower poles of the kidneys are fused in most patients via an isthmus that consists of a segment of renal parenchyma or a fibrous band. This anomaly is often asymptomatic but can be associated with urinary tract infections, ureteropelvic junction obstruction, reflux nephropathy, or stone disease. Coronal and volume-rendered images are helpful in the planning of operative stone removal, abdominal aortic aneurysm repair, or nephron-sparing renal surgery in patients with this anomaly.

History: 60-year-old male with history of gross hematuria.

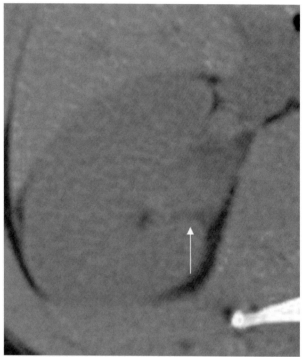

Figure 8.11   A

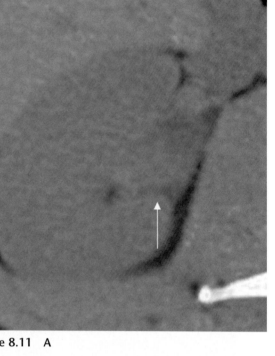

Figure 8.11   B

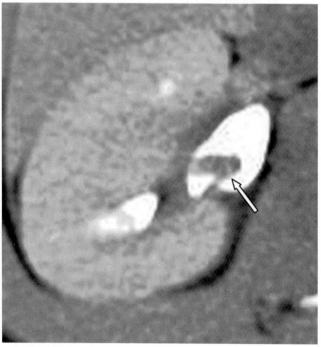

Figure 8.11   C

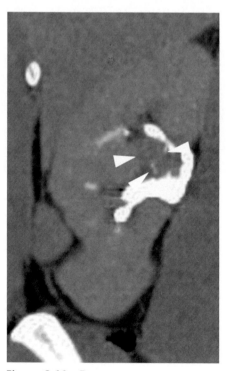

Figure 8.11   D

Findings: Axial unenhanced (A), corticomedullary phase (B), and axial and coronal excretory phase images (C, D) from a CT urogram demonstrate a 2-cm papillary mass in an upper pole infundibulum and renal pelvis of the right kidney (arrows). There are linear collections of contrast material within the central portion of the mass (arrowheads).

Diagnosis: Inverted papilloma

Discussion: Inverted papilloma is a benign renal collecting system tumor arising from transitional cell epithelium.

The CT appearance is indistinguishable from transitional cell carcinoma (TCC). Like many other tumors of transitional cell origin, the mass is papillary, frondlike, and the interstices of the mass may fill with contrast material. Inverted papillomas can recur after resection, and it is believed that they may have malignant potential. (Case courtesy of Stuart G. Silverman, M.D., Brigham and Women's Hospital, Boston, MA.)

History: 82-year-old female with hematuria before and after percutaneous ablation of a renal cell carcinoma.

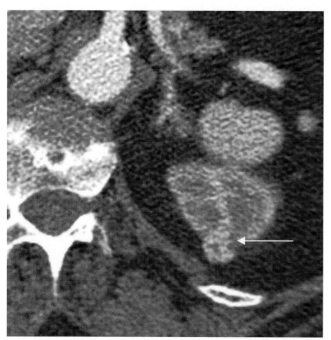

Figure 8.12   A

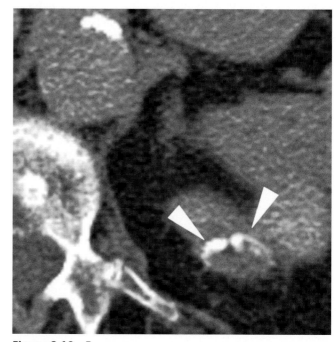

Figure 8.12   B

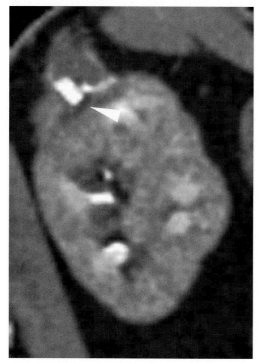

Figure 8.12   C

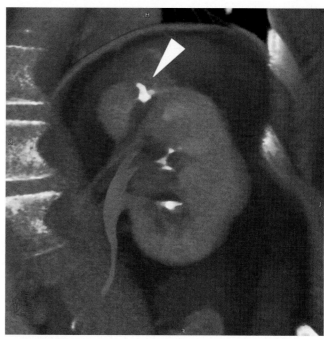

Figure 8.12   D

Findings: Contrast-enhanced axial CT image (A) demonstrates a 1.5-cm enhancing mass in the upper pole of the left kidney that was diagnosed at biopsy as a renal cell carcinoma (arrow). The tumor was treated with percutaneous radiofrequency ablation. Axial (B), coronal (C), and volume-rendered (D) images of the left kidney during the combined nephrographic/excretory phase of a CT urogram, performed using the split bolus technique, obtained 6 months after the ablation procedure demonstrate a small cavity that communicates with a distorted upper pole calyx of the left kidney (arrowheads).

Diagnosis: Post-radiofrequency ablation changes of the intrarenal collecting system with cavitation and calyceal dilatation

Discussion: Percutaneous ablation is being used with increasing frequency to treat many small renal cancers. Although data are preliminary, percutaneous ablation has been shown to be safe and effective. Hematuria often occurs following this procedure, reflecting the proximity of the treated tumor to the renal collecting system; however, it is almost always self-limited. Cavity formation may occur. Rarely, the cavity may communicate with an adjacent calyx, as in this case. Other complications are also rare and include perinephric hematoma or urinoma, both of which can be diagnosed using CT urography.

History: 41-year-old male with right flank pain and gross hematuria.

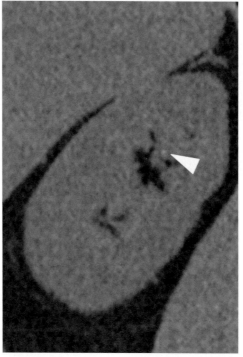

Figure 8.13 A

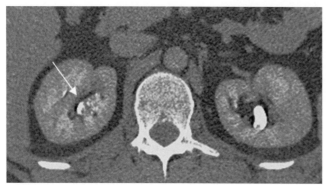

Figure 8.13 B

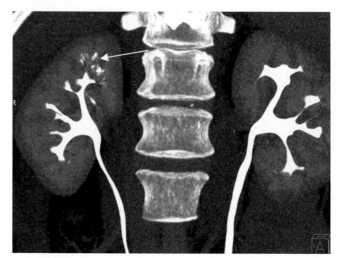

Figure 8.13 C

Findings: Unenhanced coronal image (A) and axial image obtained during combined nephrographic/excretory phase (B) of a CT urogram demonstrate an irregularly marginated stippled 1.5-cm soft tissue mass in an upper pole calyx of the right kidney (arrows) that is associated with a tiny calcification [arrowhead in (A)]. Nephrographic/excretory phase coronal maximum intensity projection image of both kidneys (C) also demonstrates the extent of the right upper pole mass.

Diagnosis: Transitional cell carcinoma of the right upper pole renal collecting system

Discussion: Seven to 10% of all kidney tumors are transitional cell carcinomas (TCCs) and 2% to 5% of TCCs are located in the upper urinary tract. Upper urinary tract TCCs most commonly present as papillary or sessile masses. The entire urothelium should be evaluated when TCC of the bladder is diagnosed; 2% to 6% of patients with bladder cancer develop synchronous or metachronous upper tract TCC. Historically, IVU has been employed to evaluate the upper tracts; however, CT urography may be used instead. CT urography is capable of detecting small upper urinary tract TCCs (see Case 8-15).

History: 55-year-old male smoker with hematuria.

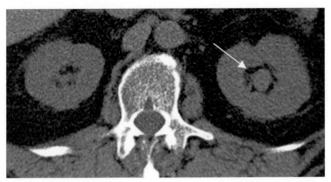

Figure 8.14   A

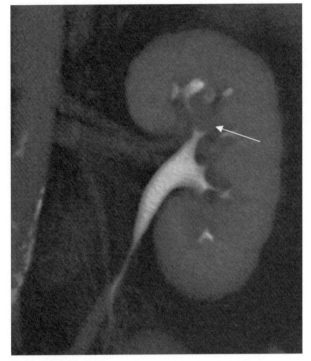

Figure 8.14   D

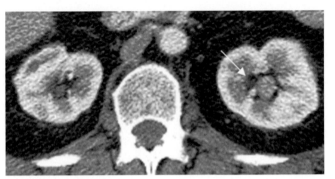

Figure 8.14   B

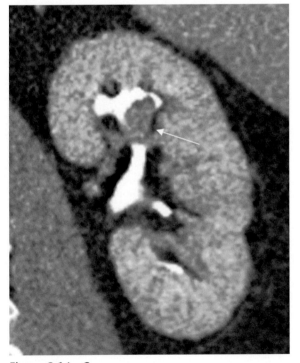

Figure 8.14   C

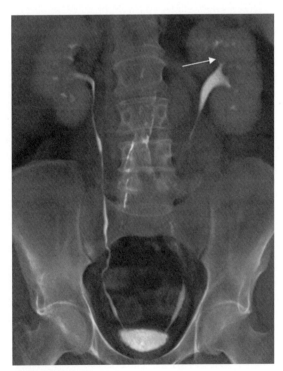

Figure 8.14   E

Findings: Axial unenhanced (A), axial corticomedullary phase (B), coronal combined nephrographic/excretory image (C), and volume-rendered images of the left kidney (D) and both kidneys (E) from a CT urogram demonstrate a noncalcified 2 × 1-cm soft tissue mass in an upper pole infundibulum of the left kidney (arrows).

Diagnosis: Noninvasive papillary transitional cell carcinoma of the upper urinary tract

Discussion: The standard differential diagnosis for a filling defect on IVU includes stone material, blood clot, and transitional cell carcinoma (TCC). Unlike conventional IVU, CT urography can be used to differentiate stones and blood clots from tumors. Nearly all (>99%) stones are of much higher attenuation on CT than are clots and tumors. Furthermore, many blood clots have higher attenuation than tumors (measuring up to 60 to 80 HU on unenhanced images rather than 30 to 40 HU). Blood clots are also entirely intraluminal and typically smoothly marginated. Tumors arise from the mucosa and are irregularly marginated, as in this case.

History: 67-year-old male with history of gross hematuria.

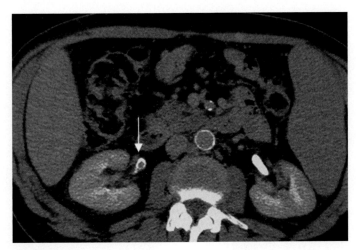

Figure 8.15

Findings: Axial image obtained during the excretory phase of a CT urogram demonstrates a 5-mm noncalcified polypoid mass (arrow) in the right renal pelvis.

Diagnosis: Upper urinary tract transitional cell carcinoma

Discussion: Detection of a small (<1 cm) transitional cell carcinoma (TCC) of the urinary tract requires careful evaluation of the collecting systems for small masslike filling defects, as in this case. Detection of early stage (noninvasive) TCC is associated with an excellent 5-year survival (>80%). Upper tract TCC may be staged with an accuracy of 85% using multidetector CT. When a low-stage TCC is identified at CT urography, anticipated treatment can be modified, with surgical approaches less aggressive than nephroureterectomy (the classic definitive surgical procedure) considered.

History: 42-year-old male with metastatic transitional cell carcinoma.

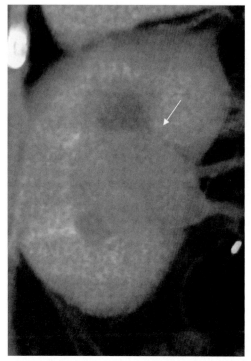

Figure 8.16   A

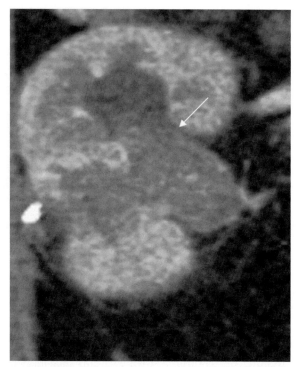

Figure 8.16   B

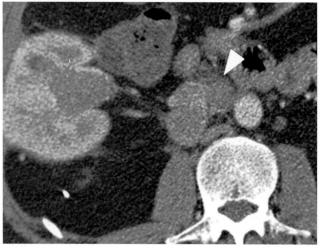

Figure 8.16   C

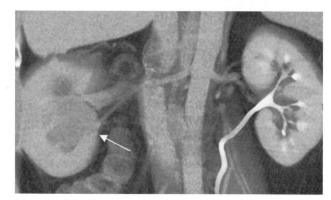

Figure 8.16   D

Findings: Coronal volume-rendered unenhanced image (A) and corticomedullary phase (B) image of the right kidney from a CT urogram demonstrate moderate hydronephrosis and a large 3.5 × 5-cm soft tissue mass in the central right renal pelvis (arrows). Axial corticomedullary phase image of the right kidney (C) demonstrates an enlarged 2-cm lymph node in the retroperitoneum (arrowhead). Volume-rendered combined nephrographic/excretory phase image of both kidneys (D) shows the large right renal mass (arrow) and a normal left kidney.

Diagnosis: Transitional cell carcinoma of the right renal pelvis with retroperitoneal lymph node metastasis

Discussion: Unlike conventional intravenous urography, CT urography evaluates extraurinary structures. The most common sites of metastatic disease from transitional cell carcinoma (TCC) of the upper urinary tract are adjacent lymph nodes, the liver, the lung, and the bones. Metastatic TCC of the upper urinary tract is associated with a poor prognosis.

CASE 8-17

History: 55-year-old male with fever and flank pain.

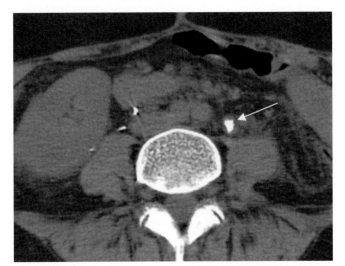

Figure 8.17 A

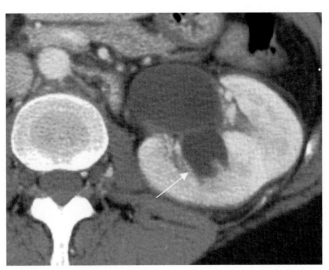

Figure 8.17 B

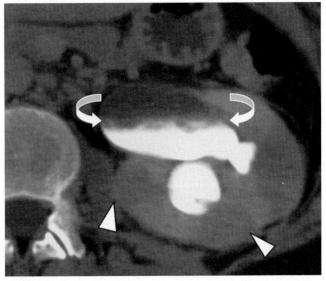

Figure 8.17 C

Findings: Unenhanced axial image (A) demonstrates a calculus in the left mid ureter (arrow). Axial images obtained during the corticomedullary (B) and excretory (C) phases of a CT urogram demonstrate moderate left pyelocaliectasis (arrow) and a fluid-debris level (curved arrows) in the dilated left intrarenal collecting system, as well as wedge-shaped areas of low attenuation in the renal parenchyma (arrowheads).

Diagnosis: Obstructed upper urinary tract with inflammatory debris and pyelonephritis

Discussion: CT urography is the optimal imaging evaluation for the primary causes and complications of urinary tract obstruction. Obstructive urolithiasis is detected on unenhanced CT alone with a sensitivity and specificity approximating 100%. However, some complications of urinary tract obstruction, such as pyelonephritis, perirenal and intrarenal abscesses, and inflammatory debris within the renal collecting system, may not be identified. CT urography can detect all these abnormalities.

History: 66-year-old female with fever and flank pain.

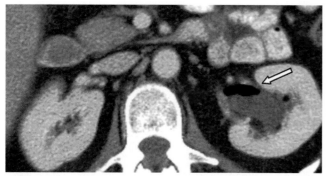

Figure 8.18   A

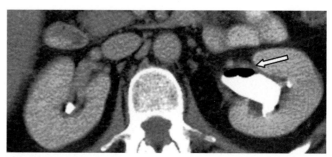

Figure 8.18   B

Findings: Axial images in the nephrographic (A) and excretory (B) phases of a CT urogram demonstrate gas within the left intrarenal collecting system (arrows).

Diagnosis: Emphysematous pyelitis (see Case 6-7)

Discussion: Gas within the intrarenal collecting system is due to four causes: prior trauma or instrumentation (e.g., cystoscopy or bladder catheterization), postoperative communication (e.g., ureterosigmoid conduit), fistulous communication (e.g., colovesical fistula), or infection with gas-forming organisms (e.g., *Escherichia coli*, *Klebsiella*

pneumoniae, *Aerobacter aerogenes*, and *Proteus mirabilis*), as seen in this case. Infection within the collecting system (emphysematous pyelitis) can be differentiated from gas-forming infection within the renal parenchyma (emphysematous pyelonephritis) using CT. Emphysematous pyelitis typically responds well to appropriate antimicrobial therapy. CT urography can be helpful in evaluating causes of gas in the intrarenal collecting system and can be used to exclude collecting system communication with a hollow viscus (e.g., colovesical fistula).

History: Paraplegic 41-year-old male with spina bifida, stone disease, and flank pain.

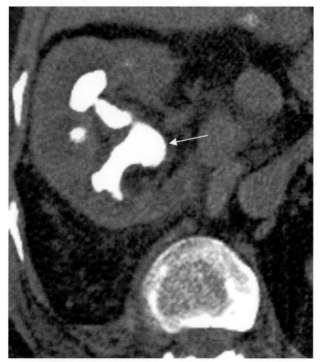

Figure 8.19   A

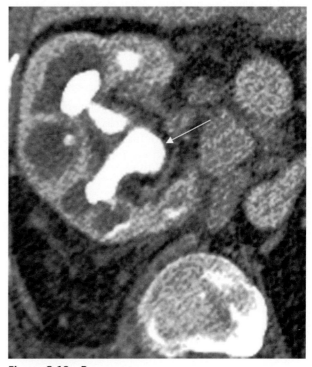

Figure 8.19   B

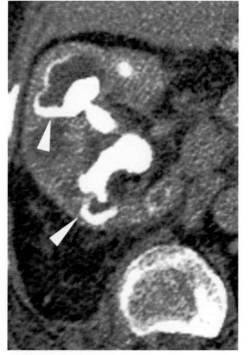

Figure 8.19   C

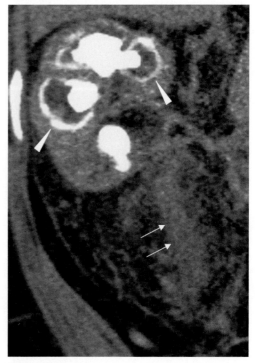

Figure 8.19   D

CASE 8-19, *continued*

Findings: Axial unenhanced (A) and corticomedullary (B) images of a CT urogram demonstrate a large branching (staghorn) calculus (arrows). Axial (C) and coronal (D) excretory phase images demonstrate lacunae surrounding multiple papillae within the renal sinus (arrowheads) and perinephric inflammatory changes surrounding the proximal right ureter (arrows).

Diagnosis: Xanthogranulomatous pyelonephritis

Discussion: Xanthogranulomatous pyelonephritis is a severe form of chronic renal parenchymal infection that often results from focal or diffuse replacement of renal parenchyma with granulomatous tissue (see Cases 5-15 and 6-14). Patients often present with flank pain, fever, or sepsis. The kidney may be enlarged and nonfunctioning, with severe caliceal deformity, urolithiasis, and hydronephrosis. CT urography is useful for demonstration of urolithiasis, inflammatory changes, as well as the papillary lacunae associated with chronic urinary tract obstruction. Lacunae have been described in patients with chronic urinary obstruction as spaces within the renal papillae that communicate with the fornices of the calyces and opacify on excretory phase imaging. Xanthogranulomatous pyelonephritis is treated typically with nephrectomy.

SUGGESTED READINGS

1. Atta MG, Whelton A. Acute renal papillary necrosis induced by ibuprofen. *Am J Ther.* 1997;4:55–60.

2. Browne RFJ, Meehan CP, Colville J, et al. Transitional cell carcinoma of the upper urinary tract: spectrum of imaging findings. *Radiographics.* 2005;25:1609–1627.

3. Dyer RB, Chen MY, Zagoria RJ. Intravenous urography: technique and interpretation. *Radiographics.* 2001;21:799–821.

4. Farrell MA, Charboneau WJ, DiMarco DS, et al. Imaging-guided radiofrequency ablation of solid renal tumors. *Am J Roentgenol.* 2003;180:1509–1513.

5. Fritz GA, Schoellnast H, Deutschmann HA, et al. Multiphasic multi-detector-row CT (MDCT) in detection and staging of transitional cell carcinomas of the upper urinary tract. *Eur Radiol.* 2006;1–9.

6. Kenney PJ. CT evaluation of urinary lithiasis. *Radiol Clin North Am.* 2003;41:979–999.

7. Kim JK, Cho KS. CT urography and virtual endoscopy: promising imaging modalities for urinary tract evaluation. *Br J Radiol.* 2003;76:199–209.

8. Noroozian M, Cohan RH, Caoili EM, et al. Multislice CT urography: state of the art. *Br J Radiol.* 2004;77:S74–S86.

9. Perlman ES, Rosenfield AT, Wexler JS, et al. CT urography in the evaluation of urinary tract disease. *J Comput Assist Tomogr.* 1996;20:620–626.

10. Rhim H, Dodd GD III, Chintapalli KN, et al. Radiofrequency thermal ablation of abdominal tumors: lessons learned from complications. *Radiographics.* 2004;24:41–52.

11. Rodriguez de Velasquez A, Yoder IC, Velasquez PA, et al. Imaging the effects of diabetes on the genitourinary system. *Radiographics.* 1995;15:1051–1068.

12. Sekine H, Mine M, Ohya K, et al. Renal papillary necrosis caused by urinary calculus-induced obstruction alone. *Urol Int.* 1995;54:112–114.

13. Torres V, Malek RS, Svensson JP. Vesicoureteral reflux in the adult: nephropathy, hypertension, and stones. *J Urol.* 1983;130:41–44.

14. Torres V, Velosa J, Holley KE, et al. The progression of vesicoureteral reflux nephropathy. *Ann Intern Med.* 1980;92:776–784.

15. Nemeth AJ, Patel SK. Pyelovenous backflow seen on CT urography. *Am J Roentgenol.* 2004;182:532–533.

16. Roy C, Pfleger DD, Tuchmann CM, et al. Emphysematous pyelitis: findings in five patients. *Radiology.* 2001;218:647–650.

17. Talner LB, Webb JA, Dail DH. Lacunae: a urographic finding in chronic obstructive uropathy. *Am J Roentgenol.* 1991;156(5):985–988.

18. Zorzos I, Moutzouris V, Korakianitis G, et al. Analysis of 39 cases of xanthogranulomatous pyelonephritis with emphasis on CT findings. *Scan J Urol Nephrol.* 2003;37(4):342–347.

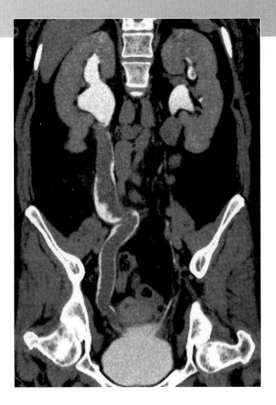

History: 60-year-old male with gross hematuria.

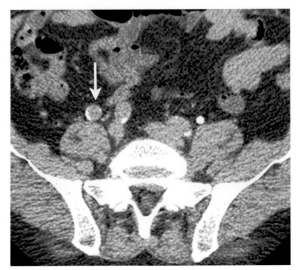

Figure 9.1   A

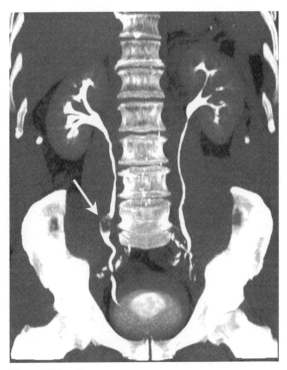

Figure 9.1   B

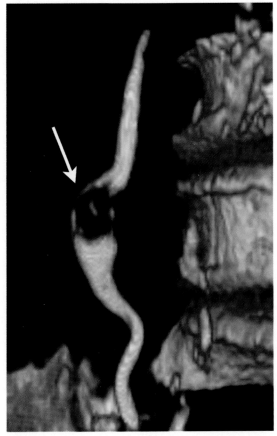

Figure 9.1   C

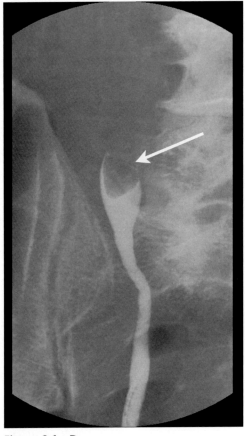

Figure 9.1   D

Findings: Axial excretory phase image (A) obtained during a CT urogram demonstrates a soft tissue mass (arrow) filling most of the lumen of the mid right ureter just lateral to the proximal right common iliac artery. Maximum intensity projection (B) and volume-rendered (C) images show that the ureteral mass (arrows) is both polypoid and stippled in appearance. There is minimal, if any, hydronephrosis and hydroureter. On an image from a retrograde pyelogram (D), the distal portion of the mass appears as a large filling defect (arrow) protruding into the dilated portion of the adjacent ureter.

Diagnosis: Transitional cell carcinoma of the ureter

Discussion: Transitional cell carcinoma (TCC) may present as a polypoid mass that arises from a portion of the ureteral mucosa and slowly grows over time. As the tumor grows, the tumor extends into and expands the lumen of the ureter. Consequently, there is little obstruction, if any. As a result, the ureter both above and below the tumor is widened. In cases of ureteral calculi, clots, and fungus balls, the distal ureter is typically narrowed. TCC can be further differentiated from other entities because TCC typically enhances after contrast material administration. On images obtained with retrograde pyelography, the widened ureter distal to the tumor and the interface of the contrast material with the tumor has been called the "goblet sign." CT urography can be helpful in defining TCC size, location, and extent. In this case, the reformatted images clearly depict the upper and lower extent of the tumor. This case was treated by local surgical excision.

CASE 9-2

History: 56-year-old female with microscopic hematuria.

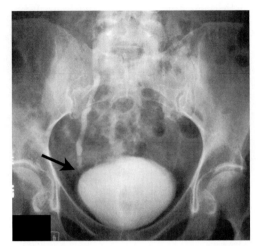

Figure 9.2   A

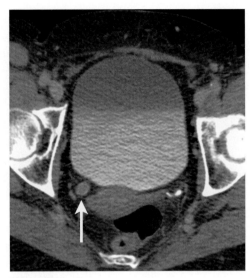

Figure 9.2   B

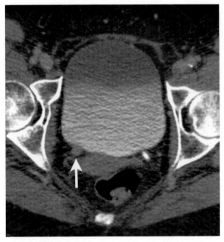

Figure 9.2   C

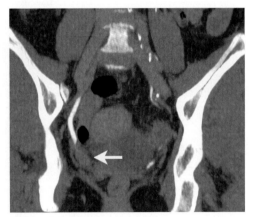

Figure 9.2   D

Findings: On an image from an intravenous urogram (A), obtained 15 minutes post injection of intravenous contrast material, the right ureter is wider than the left. Bowel gas overlies the distal right ureter, which may contain a small filling defect (arrow). Axial images (B, C) from the excretory phase of a CT urogram show a soft tissue mass (arrows) in the distal right ureter with a thin rim of contrast around its periphery (A). An oblique coronal image (D) demonstrates the upper and lower extent of the large soft tissue mass (arrow) extending close to the ureterovesical junction.

Diagnosis: Transitional cell carcinoma of the ureter

Discussion: As previously stated, most urothelial neoplasms originate in the bladder; however, they may occur anywhere where there is urothelium. When the ureter is involved, most tumors are located in the distal ureter. Overall, approximately 73% of ureteral tumors are located in the distal ureter, 24% in the middle ureter, and only 3% in the proximal ureter. This patient underwent a distal right ureterectomy. This case illustrates an advantage of CT urography relative to IVU in detecting urothelial tumors. On the IVU image, the transitional cell carcinoma (TCC) is not visualized in its entirety, in part because the distal right ureter is obscured by the overlying bladder. With CT urography, overlying structures, including the bladder, bowel gas, and bones, do not interfere with the evaluation of the ureters.

History: 77-year-old male status post transurethral resection of transitional cell carcinoma of the bladder.

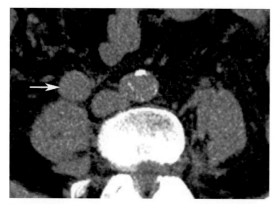

Figure 9.3   A

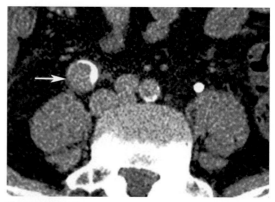

Figure 9.3   B

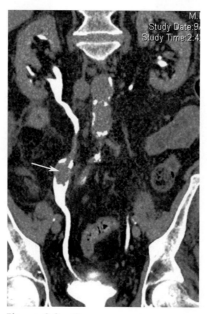

Figure 9.3   C

Findings: Axial unenhanced (A) and excretory (B) phase images from a CT urogram demonstrate a 2 × 2-cm enhancing soft tissue mass (arrows) in the mid right ureter. The mass measured 29 HU on the unenhanced images and 59 HU on the excretory phase images. Contrast material is present along the periphery of the ureter. Curved planar reformatted image (C) illustrates that the mass (arrow) is pedunculated and involves a 6-cm segment of right ureter.

Diagnosis: Papillary urothelial carcinoma

Discussion: Upper urinary tract transitional cell carcinoma (TCC) occurs in 2% to 4% of patients with bladder cancer. Approximately one-third to three-fourths of patients with upper tract TCC have bladder tumors at some time. Several reasons have been proposed to explain the low incidence of subsequent upper tract tumors in patients with bladder cancer, including the larger surface area of the bladder, downstream seeding of tumor cells, and the fact that the bladder mucosa is exposed to carcinogens for a longer duration because it acts as a reservoir. Exposure to a variety of noxious stimuli, such as cigarette smoke, phenacetin, dyes, and cyclophosphamide, is associated with an increased risk of development of urothelial metaplasia and neoplasia. TCCs of the upper urinary tract are divided into papillary (≥85%) and nonpapillary (the remainder) types. TCC occurs typically in patients 60 years or older. Males are affected more than females, and most present with hematuria. Dysuria and frequency occur more frequently with ureteral tumors. Upper tract tumors are frequently found during the workup of bladder cancers. TCC should be differentiated from benign lesions such as fibroepithelial polyps (see Case 9-17) and blood clots (see Case 9-19). (Case courtesy of Lisa Zorn, MD, and Stuart G. Silverman, MD, Brigham and Women's Hospital, Boston, MA.)

CASE 9-4

History: 56-year-old female with gross hematuria status post radical hysterectomy and radiotherapy for cervical carcinoma 9 years ago.

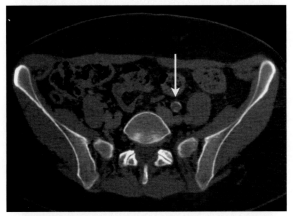

Figure 9.4 A

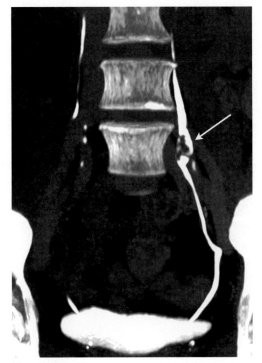

Figure 9.4 B

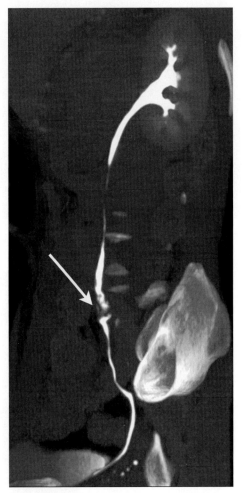

Figure 9.4 C

Findings: Axial excretory phase image (A) obtained during CT urography shows a polypoid soft tissue mass (arrow) in the left ureter. Coronal maximum intensity projection image (B) and sagittal thick-slab maximum intensity projection image (C) also show the lesion (arrows). Thin internal streaks of excreted contrast material extend into the mass. The remainder of the ureter is normal.

Diagnosis: Transitional cell carcinoma of the ureter

Discussion: This case illustrates another example of a transitional cell carcinoma (TCC) presenting as a polypoid soft tissue mass (see Cases 9-1 and 9-3). In this case, the papillary nature of the mass can be suspected since some of the excreted contrast material extends into the interstices of the mass. Ureteroscopy and biopsy were performed for histological confirmation of the diagnosis. CT urography was helpful in identifying the tumor, delineating its extent, and excluding other urothelial lesions.

History: 77-year-old female with gross hematuria.

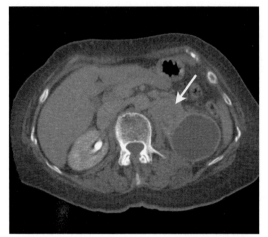

Figure 9.5   A

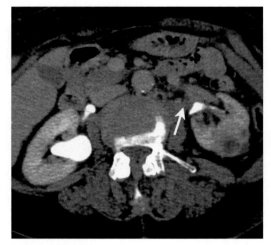

Figure 9.5   B

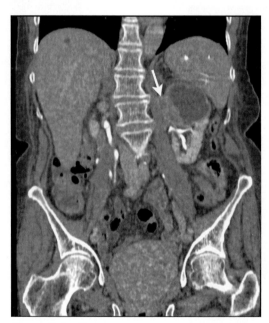

Figure 9.5   C

Findings: Axial image from the excretory phase of a CT urogram, obtained at the level of the kidneys (A), shows a hydronephrotic upper moiety of a duplex left renal collecting system. There is also a soft tissue mass (arrow) in the proximal ureter of the upper moiety. Axial image obtained at a more caudal location (B) demonstrates abnormal soft tissue (arrow) medial to the lower pole moiety renal collecting system. Low-attenuation areas along the lateral aspect of the kidney represent the inferior extent of the dilated upper pole renal collecting system. Coronal maximum intensity projection image (C) displays the dilated upper pole moiety renal collecting system and the soft tissue tumor mass (arrow) involving the upper pole moiety ureter.

Diagnosis: Transitional cell carcinoma in an upper pole ureter of a duplex collecting system

Discussion: In the past, patients with hematuria were frequently assessed with intravenous urography and/or ultrasound. When these studies did not show a cause for hematuria, conventional CT or MRI was performed. CT urography alone is often sufficient in patients with hematuria. In this patient, a large infiltrative transitional cell carcinoma (TCC) was both diagnosed and staged with CT urography. In addition to the urothelial mass, enlarged para-aortic lymph nodes and pulmonary metastases were identified.

History: 80-year-old male with carcinoma of the colon and hydronephrosis. Retrograde pyelography could not be performed due to inability to pass the cystoscope into the bladder secondary to hypospadias.

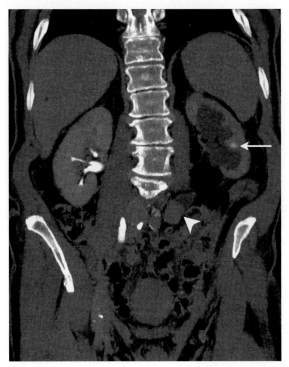

Figure 9.6   A

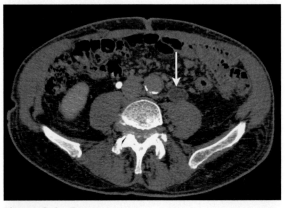

Figure 9.6   B

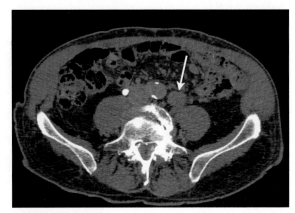

Figure 9.6   C

Findings: Coronal image (A) from the excretory phase of a CT urogram shows left-sided hydronephrosis with atrophy of the renal parenchyma. At 15 minutes after intravenous contrast material injection, there is only a tiny amount of excreted contrast in the left renal collecting system (arrow). A soft tissue density mass (arrowhead) in the dilated mid left ureter is detected in part because it is demarcated by the natural contrast between the urine and the mass. Axial excretory phase image just proximal to the mass (B) demonstrates marked dilatation of the unopacified mid left ureter (arrow). Axial phase excretory phase image obtained slightly more caudally (C) shows the large obstructing ureteral mass (arrow).

Diagnosis: Transitional cell carcinoma of the ureter

Discussion: With IVU, obstructing transitional cell carcinoma (TCC) may be difficult to diagnose. In the setting of high-grade obstruction, excretion is often delayed markedly. IVU is frequently nondiagnostic because the ureter is not opacified and therefore not visualized. With CT urography, when ureteral obstruction is present, urothelial tumors are usually detected even though the urinary tract may not be opacified at the time that the excretory phase images are obtained. The neoplasm is visible because its attenuation is higher than the adjacent unopacified urine. When the urinary tract is not opacified, the entire intrarenal collecting system and ureter should be searched carefully for portions that are of soft tissue attenuation. Urothelial masses may also be detected if early nephrographic phase images include the ureters. TCC typically enhances after contrast material administration (see Case 9-1). Therefore, the attenuation will be even higher and contrast between the enhancing tumor and the unopacified urine even more pronounced. This case shows that CT urography can be used to visualize the dilated unopacified ureter, the urothelium, and the tumor, and that CT urography can be used to diagnose urothelial neoplasms even when IVU is nondiagnostic. Furthermore, in this case, retrograde pyelography was technically not possible.

History: 79-year-old female with gross hematuria for 2 months.

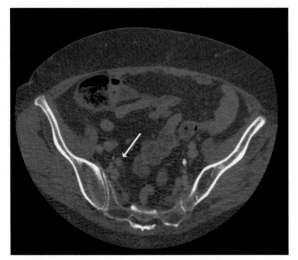

Figure 9.7   A

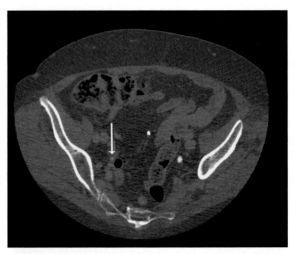

Figure 9.7   B

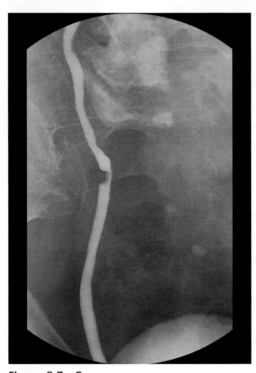

Figure 9.7   C

Findings: Axial image (A) from the excretory phase of a CT urogram shows that the lower right ureter is enlarged slightly but unopacified (arrow). Comparison can be made with the opacified normal caliber lower left ureter. Axial image obtained at a slightly more caudal level (B) demonstrates only minimal right ureteral opacification (arrow). A discrete filling defect can be seen in the right ureter at this level on a fluoroscopic spot film obtained during retrograde pyelography (C).

Diagnosis: Transitional cell carcinoma of the ureter

Discussion: Detection of intrarenal collecting system and ureteral neoplasms with CT urography is frequently dependent on differences in attenuation between the tumor and adjacent high-attenuation opacified urine. However, the ureters may not be fully opacified when excretory phase images are obtained, either as a result of obstruction (which produces delayed excretion) or due to ureteral peristalsis in an unobstructed system. When obstruction is responsible for nonopacification, renal collecting system and ureteral tumors can often be detected because there is resulting hydronephrosis and hydroureter. In these instances, the soft tissue-attenuating tumor is outlined by the water-attenuating unopacified urine in the distended urinary tract. However, if the collecting system and ureter are not opacified, and not dilated, detection of small neoplasms can be difficult. In this case, only the slight dilatation of the right ureter suggests that an abnormality is present. This case demonstrates that if the ureter is not completely opacified during CT urography, it should be followed carefully to look for any focal dilatation. In some cases, additional images or retrograde pyelography may be needed. In this patient, a polypoid right ureteral tumor was removed subsequently at ureteroscopy.

History: 77-year-old female with gross hematuria and mild right-sided hydronephrosis detected with ultrasound.

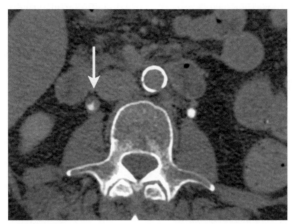

Figure 9.8   A

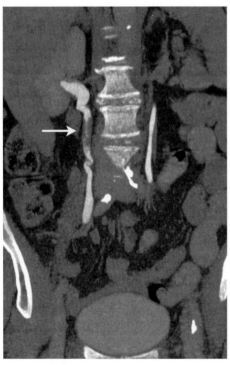

Figure 9.8   B

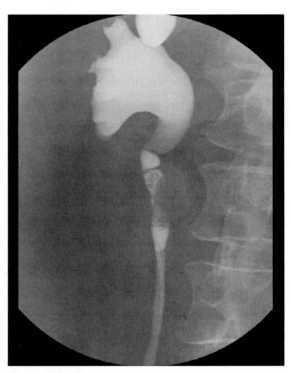

Figure 9.8   C

Findings: Axial excretory phase obtained during a CT urogram (A) shows an irregular soft tissue mass (arrow) in the anterior aspect of the proximal right ureter. Coronal image (B) shows that the mass (arrow) involves a several-centimeter-long segment of ureter, and that the ureteral lumen engulfed by the mass is irregular. Retrograde pyelogram (C) also shows a mass with a stippled surface in the proximal right ureter and hydronephrosis.

Diagnosis: Transitional cell carcinoma of the ureter

Discussion: CT urography can be used to demonstrate the surface of sessile transitional cell carcinoma (TCC) almost as well as retrograde pyelography. The interstices of the surface of sessile, papillary TCC fill with contrast material. The spatial resolution of CT urography using multidetector CT scanners is adequate enough to display these subtle changes. Unlike retrograde pyelography, CT urography can also be used to show the extent to which the ureteral wall is thickened and the extent to which the periureteral fat is involved, if at all. CT urography also allows the remainder of the urothelium to be searched for synchronous tumors. This case was treated with nephroureterectomy. The extent of tumor noted at surgery correlated well with the findings at CT urography.

History: 72-year-old female with pelvic pain and right-sided hydronephrosis detected with ultrasound.

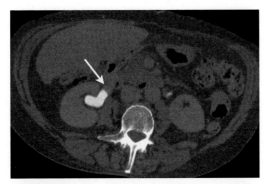

Figure 9.9 A

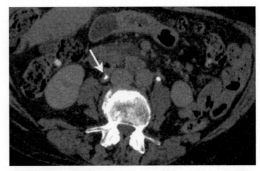

Figure 9.9 B

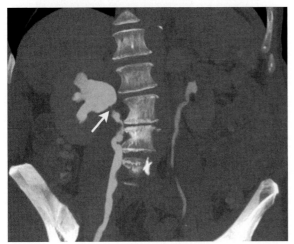

Figure 9.9 C

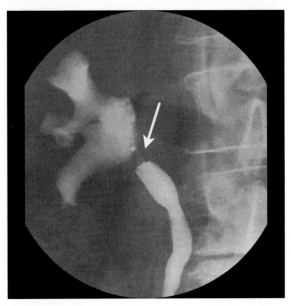

Figure 9.9 D

Findings: Axial images obtained during the excretory phase of a CT urogram at the level of the right ureteropelvic junction (A) and proximal ureter (B) show a smoothly marginated soft tissue attenuation mass (arrows) encircling the ureter, resulting in circumferential ureteral wall thickening. Coronal maximum intensity projection image (C) shows that this thickening has produced a 1-cm segment of focal narrowing of the upper ureter (arrow). Retrograde pyelogram (D) shows the same short, narrowed segment of proximal ureter (arrow).

Diagnosis: Transitional cell carcinoma of the ureter

Discussion: In rare instances (less than 1% of cases), transitional cell carcinoma (TCC) may appear as focal, circumferential ureteral wall thickening. In these cases, the tumor grows primarily along the wall of the ureter rather than into the ureteral lumen. CT urography can be used to detect both the thickened ureter, using axial images, and the narrowed ureter, best shown with three-dimensional images such as maximum intensity projection images. When the thickening is severe enough to narrow the lumen, as in this case, the findings can be detected with conventional IV urography and retrograde pyelography. Because CT urography is a cross-sectional technique, thickening can be detected in the absence of a narrowed lumen. Since CT urography does not rely on a narrowed lumen, CT urography may be more sensitive in the detection of ureteral TCC; however, this has not been confirmed in a controlled study. Circumferential wall thickening may also be secondary to inflammation, most commonly in the setting of stone disease. In most of these cases, a stone is present or there is a history of a passed stone.

History: 74-year-old male with atypical cells in the urine status post radical cystectomy for bladder cancer.

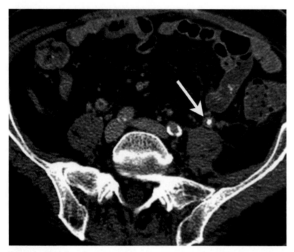

Figure 9.10   A

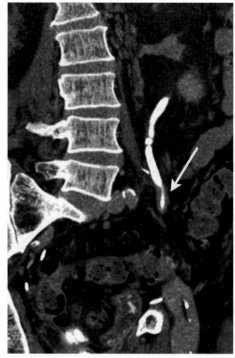

Figure 9.10   B

Findings: Axial image (A) from the excretory phase of a CT urogram shows severe circumferential thickening of the left ureteral wall (arrow). The ureteral lumen is slightly narrowed. Oblique coronal reformatted image (B) demonstrates that the ureteral wall thickening (arrow) involves a long segment of the mid left ureter.

Diagnosis: Transitional cell carcinoma of the ureter

Discussion: This case illustrates another example of transitional cell carcinoma (TCC) manifesting itself as circumferential ureteral wall thickening. Circumferential thickening can affect a long segment of ureter, as in the case illustrated here.

In some instances, the entire ureter may be involved. Because CT urography images the ureteral wall as well as the ureteral lumen, the degree of thickening and its extent can be defined. However, CT remains limited in its ability to locally stage TCC of the ureter. The depth of invasion into the muscle layer cannot be determined. Spread beyond the ureter can only be identified when it is grossly obvious. Finally, metastatic lymph nodes will only be detected when they become enlarged. (Case courtesy of Richard Cohan, MD, and Elaine Caoili, MD, University of Michigan, Ann Arbor, MI.)

History: Elderly man status post radical cystectomy and ileal loop urinary diversion for transitional cell carcinoma of the bladder with indwelling ureteral stents following treatment of superficial multifocal upper tract urothelial cancers with bacille Calmette–Guerin (BCG).

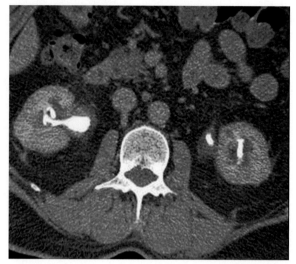

Figure 9.11   A

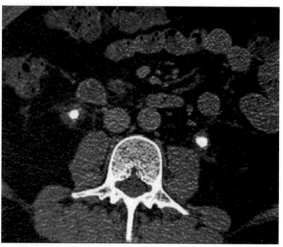

Figure 9.11   B

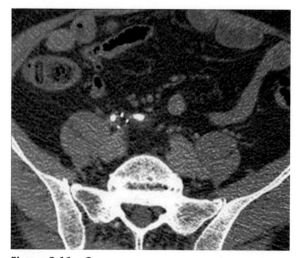

Figure 9.11   C

Findings: Axial image (A) from the excretory phase of a CT urogram demonstrates thickening of the right renal pelvic and proximal left ureteral walls. Axial image of the mid ureters (B) shows that the thickening is pronounced and extensive. The ureteral lumens are not irregular or narrowed. The thickening is still present on an axial image obtained just cephalad to the ureteroileal anastomoses (C).

Diagnosis: Diffuse urothelial wall thickening secondary to ureteral inflammation

Discussion: Diffuse urothelial wall thickening can be caused by urothelial neoplasms or ureteral inflammation, including infection. The two etiologies may have an indistinguishable CT urographic appearance, although the involvement of the entire upper tract urothelium in this case is unusual for a neoplasm, even for multifocal tumors. In this patient, there was no residual tumor. Urine cytology was negative prior to and following the CT urogram, and the ureteral thickening persisted but remained stable on follow-up studies. Superficial bladder cancers and carcinoma in situ of the bladder have been treated with topical BCG immunotherapy for years, but this agent has only rarely been used in the upper tracts. BCG is an inactive bacillus derived from *Mycobacterium bovis*. Its use in the bladder is a result of the observation in the early twentieth century that patients with tuberculosis had lower frequencies of cancers. BCG was eventually evaluated in animal and human bladders and found to successfully treat superficial bladder tumors. Currently, it is used primarily for patients with carcinoma in situ of the bladder; however, in rare instances it has also been employed in patients with bilateral upper tract disease (as in this case), patients with solitary kidneys, and patients who are not operative candidates. In this case, the severe ureteral wall thickening was likely secondary to a combination of the BCG therapy and the indwelling ureteral stents. Urothelial wall thickening may be seen in patients after BCG treatment alone and in patients with indwelling ureteral stents, although it is not usually as severe as in the case illustrated here. (Case courtesy of Richard Cohan, MD, and Elaine Caoili, MD, University of Michigan, Ann Arbor, MI.)

CASE 9-12

History: 54-year-old male with microscopic hematuria.

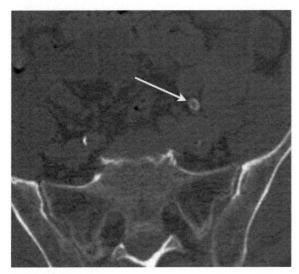

Figure 9.12 A

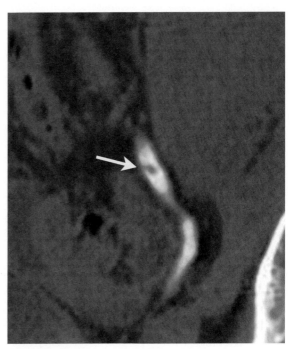

Figure 9.12 B

Findings: Axial image (A) from the excretory phase of a CT urogram shows a tiny filling defect in the mid left ureter (arrow). This filling defect is also seen on a thin-slab coronal reformatted average intensity projection image [(B), arrow].

Diagnosis: Papillary urothelial neoplasm of low malignant potential

Discussion: In 1998, the World Health Organization in conjunction with the International Society of Urological Pathology modified the terminology used to classify urothelial neoplasms. Urothelial carcinomas are divided into three groups based on their pathologic appearance: those that are high grade, those that are low grade, and those that are of the lowest grade, with this last group referred to as papillary urothelial neoplasms of low-malignant potential. These neoplasms should be differentiated from papillomas, which are benign discrete papillary growths of normally appearing urothelium that surround a central fibrovascular core.

Although the term may suggest otherwise, papillary urothelial neoplasms of low-malignant potential should be considered low-grade malignancies. Treatment is usually superficial (and performed during ureteroscopy or cystoscopy). Some patients develop recurrent disease after treatment. Recurrences may be of higher grade and may be muscle invasive. The mean interval between initial diagnosis and the detection of invasive cancer is often long, exceeding 10 years in a series reported by Cheng and associates. Thus, regular patient follow-up is required after initial therapy. This case demonstrates the ability of CT urography to detect tiny urothelial neoplasms. The tumor was only 2 or 3 mm in diameter and did not produce any luminal dilatation or irregularity. Given its location in a portion of the ureter located anterior to the sacrum, it is possible that this lesion would not have been seen on an IVU. (Case courtesy of Richard Cohan, MD, and Elaine Caoili, MD, University of Michigan, Ann Arbor, MI.)

History: 64-year-old male status post ileal loop urinary diversion with microscopic hematuria.

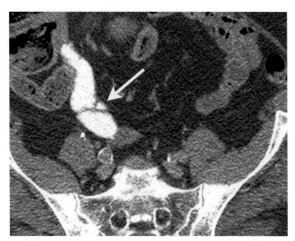

Figure 9.13   A

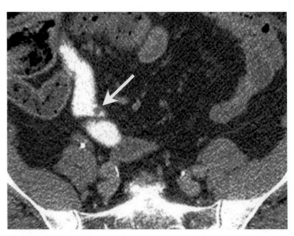

Figure 9.13   B

Findings: Axial image (A) from the excretory phase of a CT urogram obtained through the pelvis at the level of the right ureteroileal anastomosis shows a normal appearing ileal loop and a normal caliber distal right ureter (arrow). Axial image obtained slightly more caudally (B) demonstrates a tiny soft tissue nodule along the anterior aspect of the distal right ureter and just medial to the ileal loop.

Diagnosis: Transitional cell carcinoma at ureteroileal anastomosis

Discussion: Patients may develop upper tract cancers after cystectomy for transitional cell carcinoma (TCC). These can be single or multiple and can occur anywhere in the upper urinary tract. Imaging detection can be difficult when ureteral cancers develop immediately adjacent to ureteroileal anastomoses because the urothelium can appear slightly thickened in this region as a result of surgery. Furthermore, patients can develop benign strictures in this region, which may also produce symptoms. Sometimes it is necessary to evaluate the ureteroileal anastomotic regions on sequential CT urography examinations in order to determine whether distal ureteral wall thickening is due to expected postoperative changes, a benign stricture, or a new cancer. In this patient, the neoplasm, although small, is detectable because it has a round, nodular shape. (Case courtesy of Richard Cohan, MD, and Elaine Caoili, MD, University of Michigan, Ann Arbor, MI.)

History: 74-year-old male with gross hematuria. Ultrasound demonstrated left hydronephrosis. Urine cytology was positive for malignant cells. Left ureteral orifice could not be cannulated for retrograde pyelography due to inflammatory change.

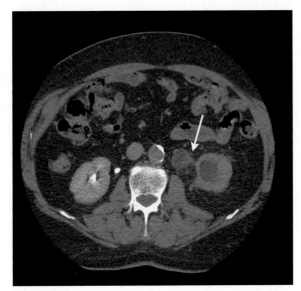

Figure 9.14 A

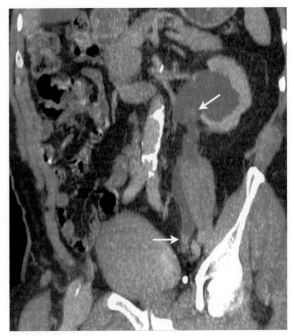

Figure 9.14 B

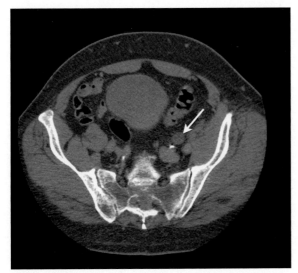

Figure 9.14 C

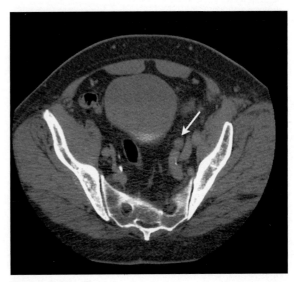

Figure 9.14 D

Findings: Axial image (A) from the excretory phase of a CT urogram demonstrates a soft tissue attenuation mass (arrow) in the medial wall of the left renal pelvis. Soft tissue stranding is noted in the adjacent perirenal fat. The left renal collecting system is dilated and not opacified due to a high-grade obstruction. Oblique coronal image (B) shows soft tissue attenuation masses (arrows) adjacent to unenhanced urine in both the upper and lower portions of the left ureter. Axial image during the excretory phase obtained just cephalad to the lower ureteral mass (C) demonstrates unopacified urine in a dilated left ureter (arrow). Axial image during the excretory phase at the level of the lower ureteral mass (D) shows that its attenuation (arrow) is higher than that of unopacified urine.

Diagnosis: Multifocal transitional cell carcinoma of the ureter

Discussion: In approximately 14% to 30% of cases, transitional cell carcinoma (TCC) is multifocal. When CT urography is performed, it is important that the entire urothelium be evaluated. This case provides another example of how ureteral neoplasms can be detected in dilated ureters, even if they do not contain opacified urine (see Case 9-6). Thus, it is not necessary to obtain additional delayed images after urinary tract excretion has occurred in these patients. This is also a case in which CT urography provided a diagnosis in a patient in whom retrograde pyelography and ureteroscopy could not be performed.

History: 62-year-old female with fever, rigors, vomiting, and right flank pain.

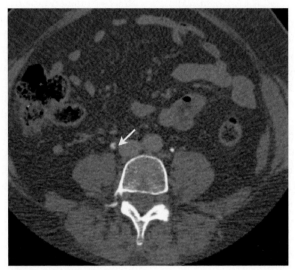

Figure 9.15 A

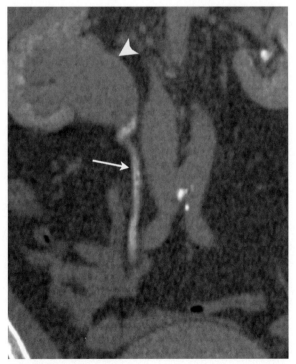

Figure 9.15 B

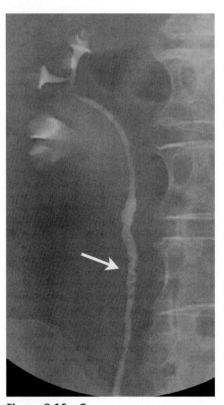

Figure 9.15 C

Findings: Axial image (A) from the excretory phase of a CT urogram shows a small filling defect (arrow) in the right ureter. Multiple similar filling defects were identified on other images. Coronal maximum intensity projection image (B) shows multiple tiny filling defects (arrow) in the opacified ureter of an upper pole moiety of a duplicated right renal collecting system. Hydronephrosis of the right lower pole moiety (arrowhead) is also seen. Fluoroscopic spot radiograph (C) from a right retrograde pyelogram of the upper moiety ureter also demonstrates multiple small filling defects (arrow).

Diagnosis: Ureteritis cystica

Discussion: Ureteritis cystica is an uncommon condition in which small cysts containing proteinaceous fluid are found in the submucosa of the ureter. When located in the intrarenal collecting system, the condition is known as pyelitis cystica; when in both locations, the term pyeloureteritis cystica is used. The etiology of the cysts is not known, but usually they are associated with stone disease and/or chronic urinary tract infection. The appearance of pyeloureteritis cystica on CT urography is similar to that on intravenous urography and retrograde pyelography. The findings are characteristic: multiple smooth, oval, mural filling defects that protrude into the collecting system or ureteral lumen. Retrograde pyelography, although used in this case, may not be needed to make a diagnosis. The imaging appearance is usually distinctive, although the differential diagnosis may also include multifocal TCCs (which are usually not as numerous), metastases (which are not uniform in shape), vascular ureteral impressions (which are almost always linear rather than ovoid), subepithelial hemorrhage (which is extremely rare), and genitourinary tuberculosis (which generally presents with other signs of tuberculous infection, such as papillary necrosis).

History: 41-year-old male with persistent microscopic hematuria, fever, left loin pain, and with previous stone passage 3 years ago, who also had known left upper moiety hydronephrosis seen on an intravenous urogram (IVU) at that time.

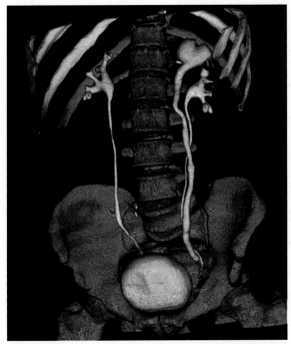

Figure 9.16   A

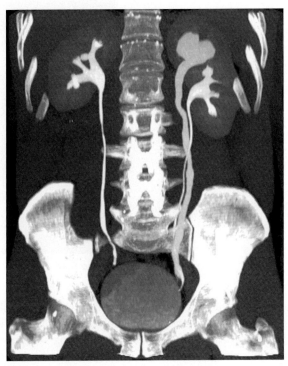

Figure 9.16   B

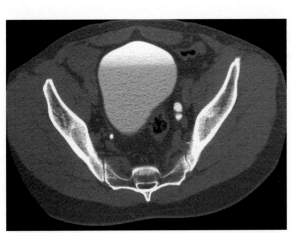

Figure 9.16   C

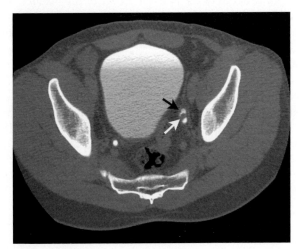

Figure 9.16   D

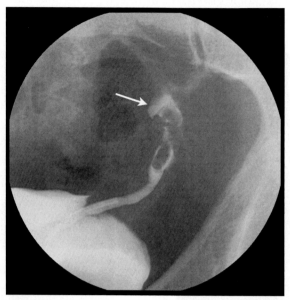

Figure 9.16   E

Findings: Volume-rendered image (A) and a thick-slab coronal maximum intensity projection image (B) from a CT urogram show a normal right renal collecting system and ureter and a duplicated left collecting system. The ureter draining the left upper pole moiety is dilated into the pelvis. Axial image obtained during the excretory phase in the prone position (C) demonstrates dependent layering of contrast material in the anterior aspect of the bladder. The single right ureter and the two left ureters (with the anterior left ureter being most dilated) are opacified with contrast material. Axial image obtained at a slightly more caudal level (D) shows irregular urothelial thickening (arrows) in the anteriorly located, left upper pole moiety, ureter. Retrograde pyelogram of the left upper pole moiety ureter (E) shows an irregular mass. The portion of the ureter distal to the filling defect demonstrates a "goblet" sign. Contrast material is seen extravasating from the ureteral lumen into the surrounding tissues (arrow), indicating that a ureteral perforation has occurred.

Diagnosis: Nephrogenic adenoma of distal aspect of a left upper moiety ureter of a duplicated urinary collecting system

Discussion: Nephrogenic adenoma or adenomatous metaplasia is a type of benign proliferation of the urothelium usually seen as a space-occupying mass in the bladder, ureter, or renal pelvis. It is associated with chronic infection or irritation, such as can occur in patients with stone disease. Nephrogenic adenoma may be solitary or multiple, papillary or sessile. Imaging cannot be used to differentiate this lesion from transitional cell carcinoma (TCC) or other benign urothelial lesions, but the histological features are characteristic. Cystoscopy or ureteroscopy and biopsy are needed to make the diagnosis.

CASE 9-17

History: 54-year-old female with gross hematuria and urinary frequency.

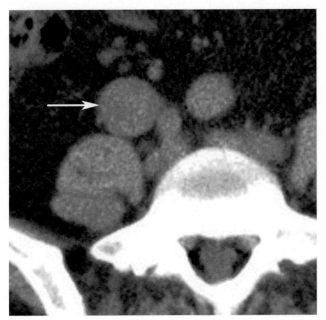

Figure 9.17   A

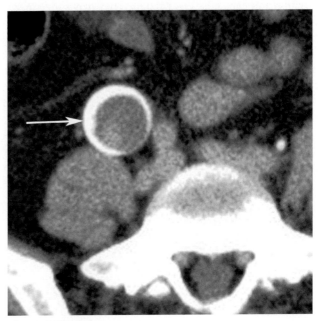

Figure 9.17   B

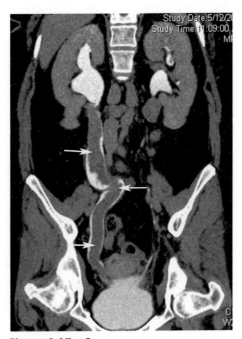

Figure 9.17   C

Findings: Axial unenhanced (A) and excretory (B) phase images from a CT urogram demonstrate a soft tissue mass within a moderately dilated right ureter. The mass enhances from 27 HU on unenhanced images to 74 HU on excretory phase images. Contrast material is seen only in the periphery of the right ureter. Curved planar reformatted image (C) illustrates the extent of the intraluminal mass (arrows), involving the entire length of a dilated right ureter.

Diagnosis: Fibroepithelial polyp

Discussion: Aside from benign papillomas, fibroepithelial polyps are the most common benign tumors of the upper urinary tract. In more than half of cases, fibroepithelial polyps occur in the upper part of the ureter or ureteropelvic junction and can cause obstruction. They may range in size from 1 to 13 cm and are frequently solitary. Composed of a core of loose fibrous tissue beneath normal urothelium, fibroepithelial polyps are usually attached by a pedicle that permits free movement of the polyp within the ureter. The etiology of fibroepithelial polyps is unknown; however, obstruction, trauma, infection, and a developmental defect have been proposed as possible causes.

Fibroepithelial polyps occur most commonly in patients younger than 40 years old, especially males. Patients may present with colicky pain and/or gross hematuria, as in this case. Because of partial obstruction, pain, which may be intermittent, is more prevalent in these tumors than in transitional cell carcinoma (TCC). Radiographically, a fibroepithelial polyp typically appears as a long, narrow, smooth filling defect. A pedicle may be present. Enhancement, demonstrated in this case, can be used to differentiate a polyp from a blood clot, which may have a similar appearance. However, fibroepithelial polyps cannot be differentiated from other polypoid urothelial cancers on the basis of imaging studies. When small, they may be resected during ureteroscopy; however, larger polyps are often removed via a nephroureterectomy, as in this case. (Case courtesy of Lisa Zorn, MD, and Stuart G. Silverman, MD, Brigham and Women's Hospital, Boston, MA.)

History: 47-year-old female with lymphoma and hematuria.

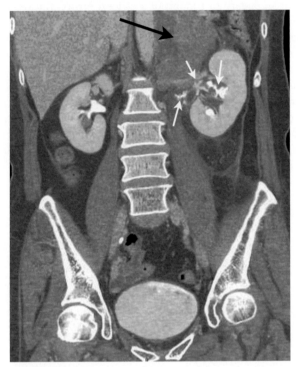

Figure 9.18 A

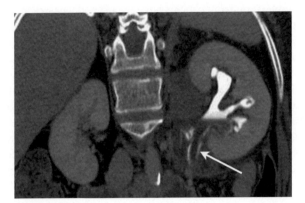

Figure 9.18 B

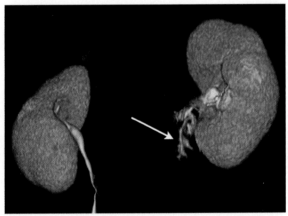

Figure 9.18 C

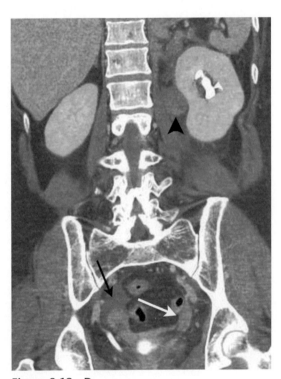

Figure 9.18 D

Findings: Coronal image (A) obtained during the combined nephrographic/excretory phase of a CT urogram using split bolus technique shows a large mass medial and superior to the left kidney (black arrow). The nephrograms are symmetric. Some excreted contrast material in the left renal sinus has an irregular shape (white arrows). Curved multiplanar coronal image (B) shows that some of the excreted contrast material outlines the proximal left ureter, which is distended and unopacified. Volume-rendered image (C) also shows extravasated contrast material in the left renal sinus and left periureteral regions (arrow). A coronal reformatted image (D) demonstrates a small soft tissue mass (white arrow) that was seen on other images to be contiguous with the dilated distal left ureter. Only a small portion of the left para-aortic soft tissue mass can be seen medial to the left kidney (arrowhead). There is a small amount of free intraperitoneal fluid in the pelvis on the right (black arrow).

Diagnosis: Lymphomatous mass obstructing the distal left ureter and producing pyelosinus backflow

Discussion: The ureter may be obstructed by both intrinsic and extrinsic processes. Although lymphoma can compress the ureters, in many patients large lymph node masses merely displace rather than obstruct the ureters. When ureteral obstruction is due to lymphoma, the ureteral involvement is almost always secondary to adjacent masses. Intrinsic primary ureteral lymphoma is rare. In this patient, the large left para-aortic mass represents extensive lymphoma. The soft tissue mass in the pelvis was also due to lymphoma, although transitional cell carcinoma should also be considered in the differential diagnosis. Pyelosinus extravasation of contrast material is most often encountered in patients with acute urinary tract obstruction. It has a characteristic appearance because it opacifies portions of the perinephric space and may fill the renal sinus and outline the ureter. It is thought to be secondary to rupture of a caliceal fornix, the weakest point in the urinary tract, usually as a result of an abrupt rise in intrarenal collecting system pressure caused by sudden obstruction. Rarely, however, it can also be identified in patients with chronic obstruction, as in this case. Beyond relieving the obstruction or diverting the urine, no additional treatment is required as long as the extravasated urine is not infected. Usually, the extravasation resolves if the obstruction is relieved, but sometimes it ceases even when the obstruction is ongoing. (Case courtesy of William Weadock, MD, University of Michigan, Ann Arbor, MI.)

History: 74-year-old female on hemodialysis for acute renal failure with gross hematuria following a renal biopsy.

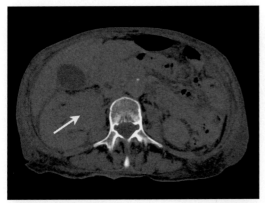

Figure 9.19   A

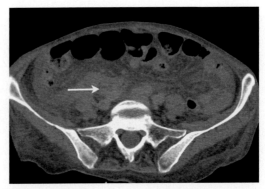

Figure 9.19   B

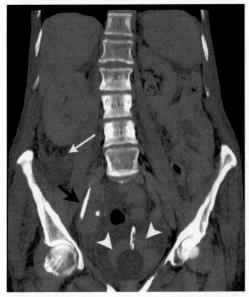

Figure 9.19   C

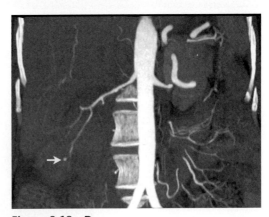

Figure 9.19   D

Findings: Unenhanced axial image from a CT urogram obtained at the level of the kidneys (A) shows homogeneous soft tissue attenuation material (arrow) in a dilated right renal collecting system and right renal pelvis. Unenhanced axial image obtained through the pelvis (B) also shows similar high-attenuation material in the right ureter (arrow) and the surrounding retroperitoneal fat. Coronal image (C) during the excretory phase shows no excretion of contrast material by either kidney, secondary to the acute renal failure. There is thickening of the right perirenal fascia and stranding in the right perinephric space (arrow). High-attenuation material is also noted in the bladder (arrowheads), surrounding the inflated balloon of a Foley catheter. A short segment of an intravenous hemodialysis catheter (black arrow) is visible in the right common iliac vein. A coronal thin-slab maximum intensity projection image obtained during subsequent CT arteriogram (D) demonstrates a tiny focal collection of contrast material in the lower pole of the right kidney.

Diagnosis: Hemorrhage from a right renal artery branch pseudoaneurysm as a result of renal biopsy

Discussion: Blood clot in the renal collecting system and ureter is of soft tissue attenuation on CT. Patients with blood clots usually have gross hematuria, so active bleeding is suspected clinically. CT urography can be used to search for possible etiologies, including infarcts, aneurysms, pseudoaneurysms, and arteriovenous malformations. However, in patients with known or suspected active hemorrhage, the protocol can be modified to include an additional series of images during the arterial phase, typically 30 seconds after contrast material injection. Unenhanced CT was useful in this case because it demonstrated the extent of the hemorrhage. The arterial phase images demonstrated the pseudoaneurysm, which was treated successfully by transcatheter embolization.

History: Elderly male with history of prostate cancer and gross hematuria.

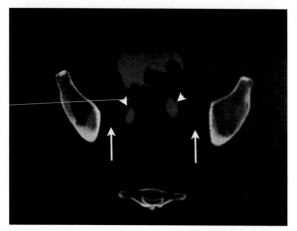

Figure 9.20   A

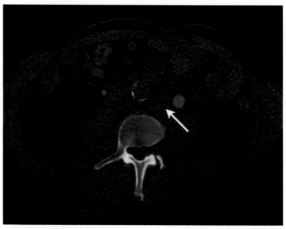

Figure 9.20   B

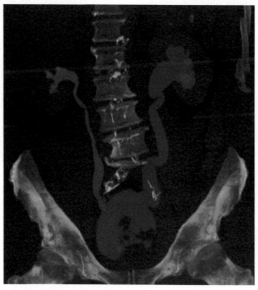

Figure 9.20   C

Findings: Axial image (A) at the level of the bladder obtained during the excretory phase of a CT urogram imaged using wide windowing demonstrates bilateral iliac lymph node enlargement (arrows) and bilateral hydroureter (arrowheads). A lobulated soft tissue mass encroaches on the bladder and narrows the distal left ureter. Axial image at the level of the abdominal aorta (B) shows an enlarged left para-aortic lymph node (arrow) and left hydroureter. Coronal thick-slab maximum intensity projection image (C) reveals bilateral hydronephrosis and hydroureter more marked on the left than the right, extending to the bladder base, where there is a large mass. Also, multiple sclerotic areas are noted in the pelvic bones.

Diagnosis: Bilateral ureteral obstruction secondary to metastatic prostate cancer

Discussion: CT urography can be used to identify different causes of hydronephrosis. Many different pelvic neoplasms may invade the bladder and distal ureters and obstruct one or both ureters. In this case, the CT urogram showed a prostate cancer invading the bladder and obstructing both ureters. In addition, CT urography revealed pelvic and retroperitoneal lymph node enlargement. In patients with hydronephrosis, the information provided by CT urography is useful to the interventional radiologist prior to percutaneous nephrostomy or stent placement in the appropriate clinical scenario. In this case, the CT urogram was used for diagnosis, tumor staging, and treatment planning.

CASE 9-21

History: Elderly male with persistent left flank pain despite passing a left ureteral stone.

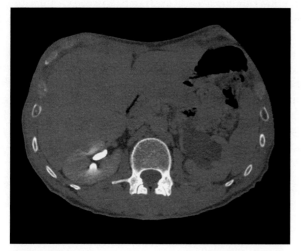

Figure 9.21   A

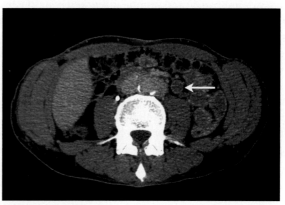

Figure 9.21   B

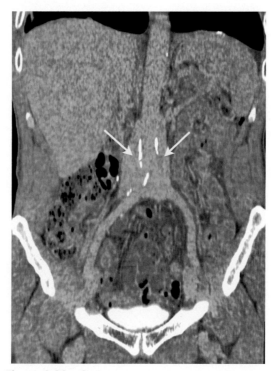

Figure 9.21   C

Findings: Excretory phase axial image from a CT urogram (A) shows severe left-sided hydronephrosis with delayed excretion into the left renal collecting system. Axial image, obtained more caudally, through the mid abdomen (B) reveals an infiltrative para-aortic soft tissue mass, a dilated nonopacified left ureter (arrow), and a normal caliber opacified right ureter. Coronal image centered at the level of the abdominal aorta (C) demonstrates the para-aortic soft tissue mass (arrows) extending to the aortic bifurcation.

Diagnosis: Primary retroperitoneal fibrosis, with encasement and obstruction of the left ureter

Discussion: Retroperitoneal fibrosis (RPF) is most prevalent between the ages of 40 and 60 years. RPF may be idiopathic in etiology (also termed primary RPF), but it may also be secondary to a variety of benign conditions, including medications (most typically, methysergide), collagen vascular disease, and abdominal aortic aneurysms. RPF may

Chapter 9: Ureters   **201**

also be caused by malignant tumors (e.g., lymphoma, prostate cancer, and breast cancer), which occasionally produce a desmoplastic and fibrotic reaction when they involve or spread to the retroperitoneum. The presentation of RPF is usually insidious. Many patients complain of poorly localized abdominal or flank pain. Gastrointestinal disturbances are common. Patients may develop weight loss, anorexia, and fever. The mean duration of symptoms prior to diagnosis is 4 months. In advanced stages, ureteral obstruction and acute renal failure may develop. On CT urography, RPF usually produces a confluent retroperitoneal soft tissue mass, typically centered at the level of the fourth lumbar vertebral body. The mass usually extends anterior and lateral to the abdominal aorta and, often, the inferior vena cava. The aorta and inferior vena cava are rarely displaced anteriorly by masses due to benign causes of RPF. This feature helps distinguish benign from malignant causes of RPF and other malignant causes of retroperitoneal lymph node enlargement since these typically encircle and elevate the aorta and inferior vena cava. Medial deviation of both ureters, which can be seen on CT urography, has been considered a classic manifestation of RPF but is often absent. Patients with RPF usually respond to immunosuppressive agents, with high-dose steroids most commonly employed.

CASE 9-22

History: 42-year-old female with chronic back pain and intermittent urinary tract infections.

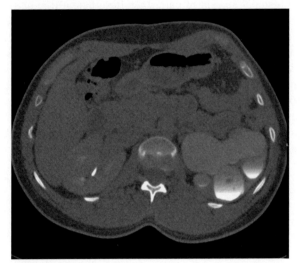

Figure 9.22   A

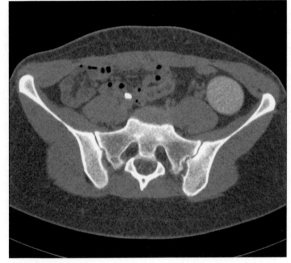

Figure 9.22   B

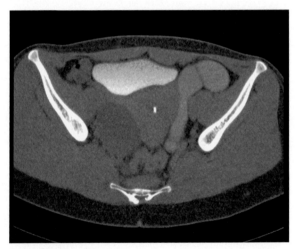

Figure 9.22   C

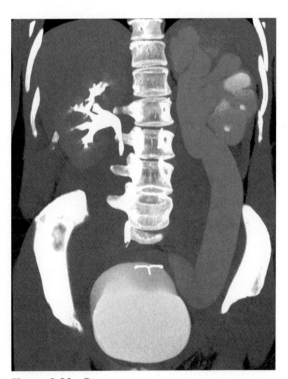

Figure 9.22   D

Findings: Axial image (A) from the excretory phase of a CT urogram shows severe left-sided hydronephrosis with layering of contrast material and debris within the collecting system. Two additional axial images (B, C) during the excretory phase demonstrate severe dilatation of the left ureter that continues into the pelvis. Coronal thick-slab maximum intensity projection image (D) shows the severe collecting system and ureteral dilatation, with the latter extending to the distal left ureter, which tapers smoothly and terminates above the level of the ureterovesical junction. An intrauterine contraceptive device is also noted.

Diagnosis: Primary megaureter

Discussion: Primary megaureter is a congenital abnormality of the urinary tract. It is usually unilateral (80% of cases) and is approximately four times more common in men. It results from neuromuscular dysfunction of a short segment of the distal-most portion of the ureter. The affected, narrowed segment is not able to peristalse and therefore does not efficiently propel urine into the bladder. Varying degrees of obstruction result. In some cases, there is marked dilatation of the proximal portions of the ureter. The ureteral segment just proximal to the aperistaltic segment is often the most dilated. In contrast to dilatation produced by other causes of urinary tract obstruction, the ureter proximal to the distal segment continues to peristalse briskly and, therefore, may change in appearance if the ureter is imaged at different times (with different segments of the ureter being more dilated). Patients with primary megaureter may be asymptomatic. When symptoms are present, they usually consist of pain, infection, hematuria, or stone disease. Treatment, if indicated, is with ureteroneocystostomy. Primary megaureter is rarely associated with congenital megacalices and congenital ureteropelvic junction obstruction. This case illustrates how coronal and maximum intensity projection images obtained at CT urography can display the marked dilatation produced by primary megaureter. CT urography can also be used to demonstrate that the ureter smoothly tapers distally just above a short segment of ureter that is normal in caliber or narrowed.

History: 51-year-old female with left flank pain, recurrent urinary tract infections, and persistent enuresis.

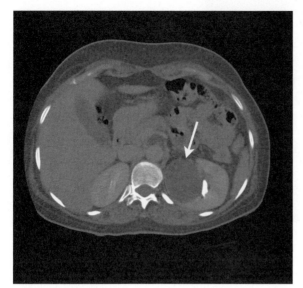

Figure 9.23   A

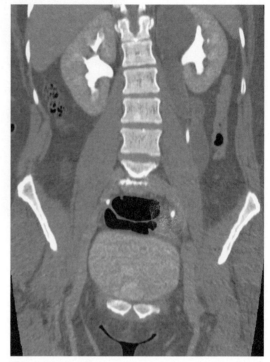

Figure 9.23   B

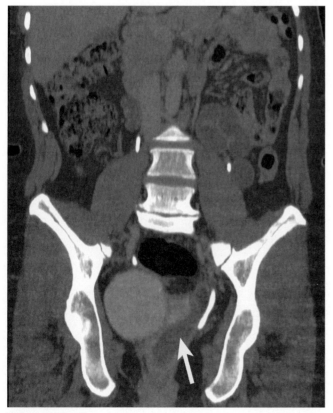

Figure 9.23   C

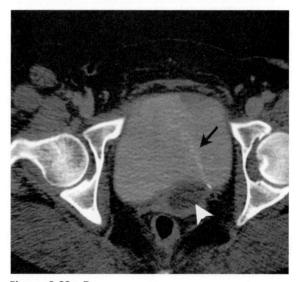

Figure 9.23   D

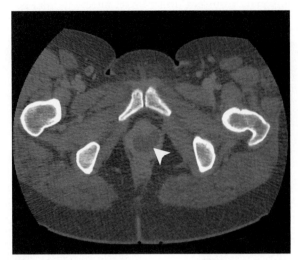

Figure 9.23   E

Findings: Axial image (A) from the excretory phase of a CT urogram shows a duplicated left-sided renal collecting system with a dilated unopacified left upper pole moiety (arrow). Coronal images (B, C) show the dilated upper pole moiety collecting system and upper pole ureter (arrow) that continues inferior to the bladder and inserts into the vagina (arrowhead). Axial excretory phase images (D, E) demonstrate a ureteral jet (arrow) from the normally inserting lower pole moiety as well as the dilated ectopically inserting upper pole moiety ureter (arrowhead).

Diagnosis: Ectopic ureterocele inserting into the vagina in a patient with a duplicated collecting system

Discussion: Ectopic ureteroceles in duplex ureters always arise from the upper pole moiety ureter. This ureter may be associated with obstruction (often related to the ureterocele), upper pole renal parenchymal dysplasia, vesicoureteral reflux, prolapse into the urethra, persistent infections, or calculi. Ectopic insertion of the ureter outside of the bladder in a woman always results in incontinence. The result of an ectopic ureter in men is different since men will still be continent as long as the ureter inserts above the external sphincter, which is at the urogenital diaphragm. Thus, males with ectopic ureters that insert into the seminal vesicles, for example, are still continent. In this case, examination under anesthesia confirmed that the ectopic ureter inserted into the vagina.

CASE 9-24

History: 47-year-old female complaining of leakage of urine from her vagina 7 days following laparoscopic myomectomy for uterine fibroids.

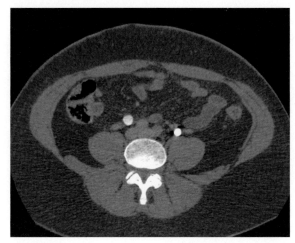

Figure 9.24 A

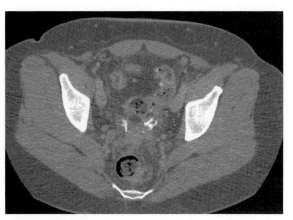

Figure 9.24 B

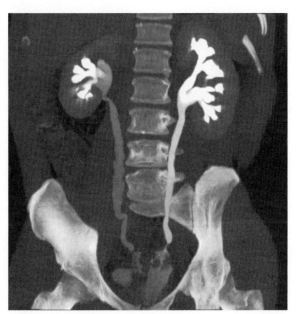

Figure 9.24 C

Findings: Axial image (A) from the excretory phase of a CT urogram shows bilateral hydroureter. On an axial image obtained through the pelvis (B) extravasated contrast material can be seen bilaterally. Coronal maximum intensity projection image (C) demonstrates bilateral ureteral dilatation proximal to contrast extravasation, which appears to be originating from both distal ureters.

Diagnosis: Bilateral iatrogenic injury of the lower ureters

Discussion: CT urography can be helpful in diagnosing ureteral injuries after surgery. Since excretory phase images are obtained, extravasation of excreted contrast material can be detected, indicating the presence of a leak. Such leaks will result in the formation of pelvic fluid collections. Other causes of postoperative fluid collections include hematomas, seromas, and lymphoceles, although in each of these cases there is no urine extravasation. Usually, hydronephrosis is not present unless there is concomitant obstruction. In this case, CT urography was helpful in delineating the site and nature of the ureteral injuries and in planning subsequent treatment. This patient was treated with right retrograde ureteral stent placement and left percutaneous nephrostomy followed by surgical reconstruction.

SUGGESTED READINGS

1. Babaian RJ, Johnson DE. Primary carcinoma of the ureter. *J Urol.* 1980;123:357–359.

2. Caoili EM, Inampudi P, Cohan RH, et al. Multidetector CT urography of upper tract urothelial neoplasms. *Am J Roentgenol.* 2005;184:1873–1881.

3. Cheng L, Neumann RM, Bostwick DG. Papillary urothelial neoplasms of low malignant potential: clinical and biologic implications. *Cancer.* 1999;86:2102–2108.

4. Elliott SP, McAninch JW. Ureteral injuries: external and iatrogenic. *Urol Clin North Am.* 2006;33:55–66.

5. Ford TF, Watson GM, Cameron KM. Adenomatous metaplasia (nephrogenic adenoma) of urothelium. An analysis of 70 cases. *Br J Urol.* 1985;57:427–433.

6. Epstein JI, Amin M, Reuter VR, et al. The World Health Organization/International Society of Urological Pathology consensus classification of urothelial (transitional cell) neoplasms of the urinary bladder. *Am J Surg.* 1998;22:1435–1448.

7. McMillin KI, Gross GH. CT demonstration of peripelvic and periureteral non-Hodgkin lymphoma. *Am J Roentgenol.* 1985;144:945–946.

8. Meyer JP, Persad R, Gillat DA. Use of bacille Calmette–Guerin in superficial bladder cancer. *Postgrad Med J.* 2002;78:449–454.

9. Nolte-Ernsting C, Cowan N. Understanding multislice CT urography techniques: many roads lead to Rome. *Eur Radiol.* September 5, 2006 [Epub ahead of print].

10. Oliva E, Young RH. Nephrogenic adenoma of the urinary tract: a review of the microscopic appearance of 80 cases with emphasis on unusual features. *Modern Pathol.* 1995;8:722–730.

11. Yokogi H, Wada Y, Mizutani M, et al. Bacillus Calmette–Guerin perfusion therapy for carcinoma in situ of the upper urinary tract. *Br J Urol.* 1996;77:676–679.

12. Yousem DM, Gatewood OM, Goldman SM, et al. Synchronous and metachronous transitional cell carcinoma of the urinary tract: prevalence, incidence, and radiographic detection. *Radiology.* 1988;167:613–618.

CHAPTER TEN

CT UROGRAPHY OF THE BLADDER

RICHARD H. COHAN, MD

ELAINE M. CAOILI, MD

JONATHON M. WILLATT, MD

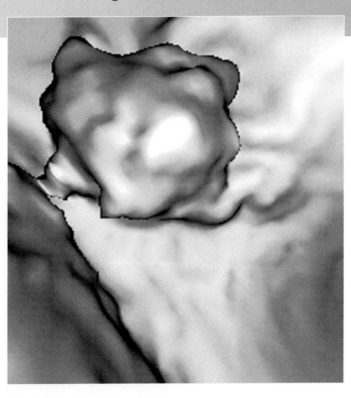

History: 62-year-old male with gross hematuria.

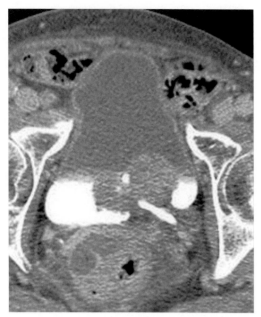

Figure 10.1   A

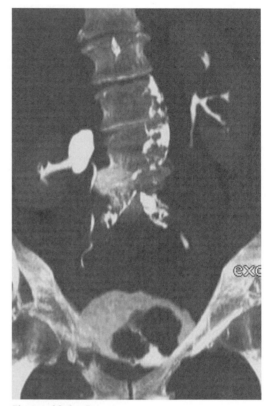

Figure 10.1   B

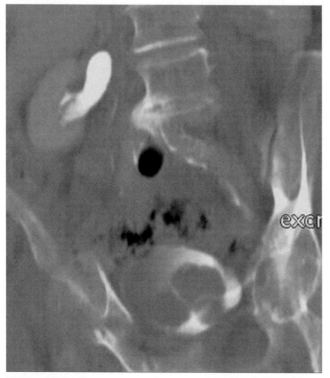

Figure 10.1   C

Findings: An excretory phase axial CT image (A) demonstrates a small amount of excreted contrast material in the bladder. The contrast material layers dependently on the right side of the bladder. A small projection of contrast material extends medially across the midline. There is a bilobed 2.5 × 4.5-cm mass along the left posterior aspect of the bladder, which surrounds the region of the left ureterovesical junction; however, the distal left ureter is not distended. The interface between the bladder and the perivesical fat is fairly smooth throughout. The maximum and average intensity projection coronal images (B, C) also demonstrate the bladder mass.

Diagnosis: Large polypoid transitional cell carcinoma

Discussion: Large urothelial neoplasms may be detected on axial CT urography images in both opacified and unopacified portions of the bladder. These masses are often, but not always, seen on three-dimensional reconstructed images. In this case, urothelial neoplasm is the most likely diagnosis, given the rounded and lobulated appearance. Occasionally, blood clot can have this morphology.

Transitional cell carcinomas are the most common bladder malignancies, accounting for 95% of bladder cancers in areas in which schistosomiasis is not endemic (in which case squamous cell carcinoma is more common). They can have flat or polypoid/papillary morphology, with the former being more difficult to detect and also more likely to be invasive. When bladder cancers are superficial, they are often treated locally. Invasive tumors are typically treated with more aggressive surgery (e.g., cystectomy and pelvic lymph node dissection). Patients with locally treated tumors should be followed closely because recurrences and/or metachronous lesions frequently develop. Although such follow-up was previously performed primarily by obtaining periodic urine cytology specimens and cystoscopy, CT urography may also play a role in monitoring these patients.

Bladder cancer staging is performed with the TNM classification system and involves assessment of the degree of muscle invasion (with superficial being T2a and deep being T2b) and involvement of the perivesical fat (T3) or adjacent pelvic organs or pelvic sidewall (T4).

History: 53-year-old male with gross hematuria.

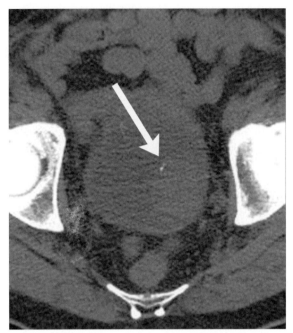

Figure 10.2   A

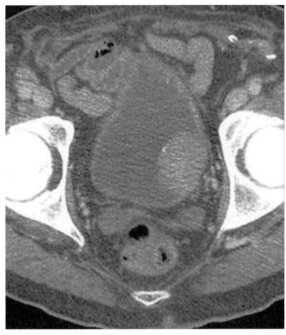

Figure 10.2   B

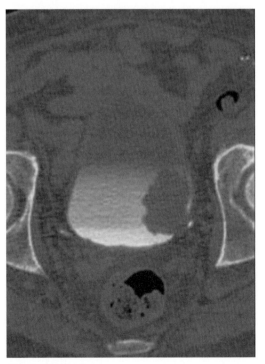

Figure 10.2   C

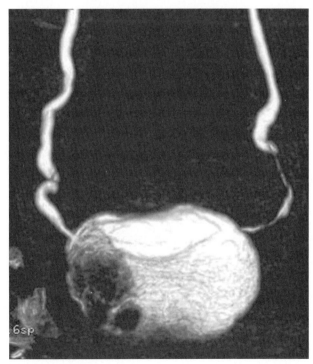

Figure 10.2   D

Findings: Unenhanced (A), nephrographic phase (B), and excretory phase (C) axial images from a CT urogram demonstrate a large 3-cm ovoid mass in the left posterolateral aspect of the bladder. The mass is visualized on images obtained during all three phases, whether outlined by unenhanced or contrast material-containing urine in the adjacent bladder lumen. There are subtle punctate calcifications (arrow) on the surface of the mass. The mass demonstrates enhancement similar to that of the bladder wall on the nephrographic phase images. A posteroanterior volume-rendered image (D) also demonstrates the mass.

Diagnosis: Transitional cell carcinoma

Discussion: The most likely diagnosis is urothelial neoplasm, with transitional cell carcinoma (TCC) being most common. Although the differential diagnosis of a large filling defect also includes blood clot and fungus ball, these diagnoses are unlikely given the presence of the tiny surface calcifications. Rarely, inflammatory processes can have focal masslike appearances. Cystoscopy is required for definitive diagnosis. This case provides an excellent illustration of how large urothelial carcinomas that have masslike configurations may be detected by CT urography even on the unenhanced images because they are well-outlined by water attenuation urine.

History: 61-year-old male with microscopic hematuria status post right nephrectomy for transitional cell carcinoma.

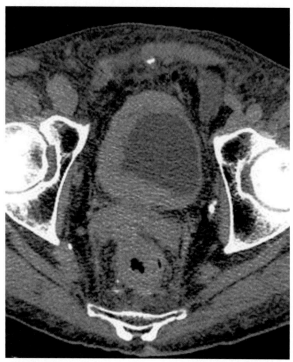

Figure 10.3   A

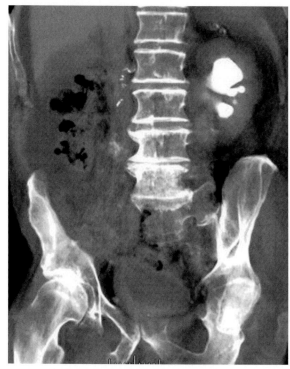

Figure 10.3   B

Findings: An excretory phase axial CT urography image (A) demonstrates extensive thickening of the right lateral and posterior wall of the bladder. Excretion of urine containing contrast material into the bladder is delayed. A thick-slab average intensity projection image (B), obtained through the anterior aspect of the bladder, also demonstrates bladder wall thickening. On this image, the thickening extends along the inferior aspect of the bladder. In addition, there is left pelvocaliectasis and an unopacified left ureter. These findings suggest that the left renal collecting system is obstructed.

Diagnosis: Transitional cell carcinoma

Discussion: In most instances, focal bladder wall thickening, as seen in this case, is due to a bladder neoplasm. Although CT cannot be used to determine depth of tumor invasion definitively, most bladder neoplasms producing this degree of wall thickening have invaded the muscular layer and are at least stage T2. Obstruction of the left renal collecting system may be due to the bladder neoplasm, which crosses the midline posteriorly to affect the left side of the bladder as well.

Cystitis can also produce bladder wall thickening but is usually diffuse. Once asymmetric bladder wall thickening is detected on CT urography, follow-up cystoscopy is warranted to allow for a definitive diagnosis.

History: 57-year-old female with positive urine cytology status post nephrectomy for transitional cell carcinoma and treatment of superficial bladder cancer.

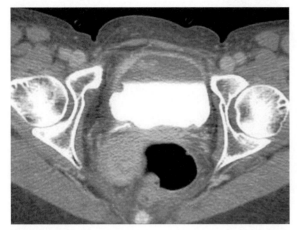

Figure 10.4   A

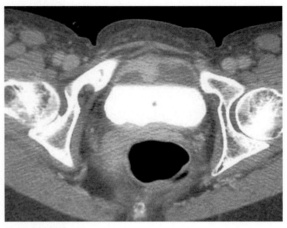

Figure 10.4   B

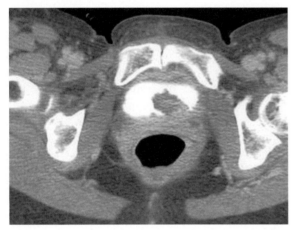

Figure 10.4   C

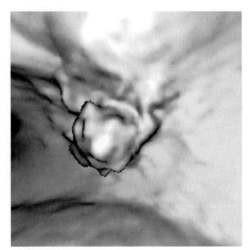

Figure 10.4   D

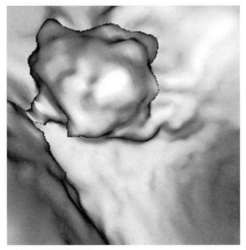

Figure 10.4   E

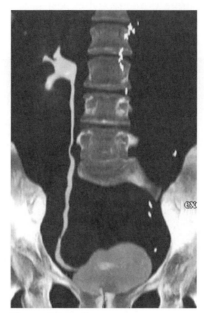

Figure 10.4 F

Findings: Three axial excretory phase CT urographic images are provided. The first (A) demonstrates asymmetric thickening of the right anterolateral bladder wall. In addition, a small mass projects medially into the anterior aspect of the opacified portion of the bladder lumen. The second axial image (B) demonstrates a small round mass projecting into the bladder lumen from the anterior wall of the bladder. This mass is seen even though it is surrounded by unopacified urine. The third axial image (C) demonstrates a lobulated mass located inferiorly at the bladder base. Two virtual cystoscopic images (D, E) demonstrate two of the masses seen on the axial images (A, C). A thick-slab maximum intensity projection image (F) does not demonstrate the two more cephalad lesions.

Diagnosis: Multifocal transitional cell carcinoma

Discussion: Urothelial neoplasms must be strongly considered as the most likely diagnoses (for the focal bladder wall thickening and the three masses) in this patient, although cystitis can occasionally produce masslike bladder abnormalities. The poorly defined intraluminal bladder abnormality located anteriorly on the right may represent a small amount of blood clot.

Up to one-third of bladder cancers are multifocal at the time of diagnosis. For this reason, it is important that the radiologist not give in to satisfaction of search. Careful attention must be paid to the remainder of the bladder once a mass is detected since other masses may be present. Also, patients with bladder cancer must be followed carefully when they are treated without bladder resection since additional cancers or recurrences may develop.

Bladder cancers may not be identified on standard three-dimensional reconstructed images. Lesions can be obscured by densely opacified urine. For this reason, one should not rely exclusively on three-dimensional images for image interpretation. Axial and/or thin section reformatted images should be carefully scrutinized in all patients.

The CT data set can be used to obtain many types of reconstructions, including virtual cystoscopic images. High-quality images can be obtained by utilizing differences in attenuation between the opacified or unopacified portions of the bladder lumen and the adjacent bladder wall or mural masses attached to the bladder wall. These images offer the urologist a view similar to that seen at cystoscopy. Although these views may serve as helpful adjuncts, they do not provide more information than the axial images.

CASE 10-5

History: 45-year-old male with gross hematuria.

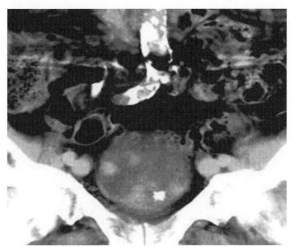

Figure 10.5   A

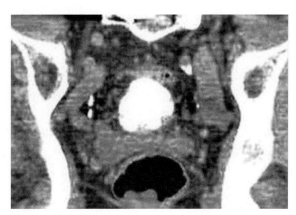

Figure 10.5   B

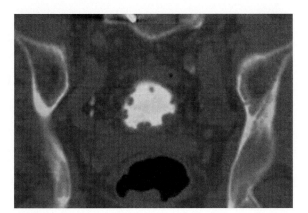

Figure 10.5   C

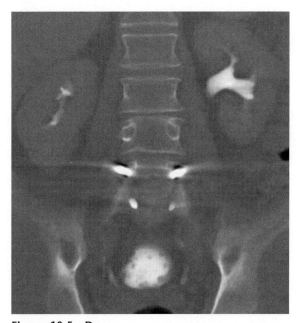

Figure 10.5   D

Findings: Two thin section (1.25 mm thick) coronal excretory phase images (A, B) are provided of the anterior and posterior aspects of the bladder using standard soft tissue windowing. The second image (B) is also shown using wide windows (C). These images demonstrate multiple mural masses projecting into the bladder lumen. The masses are easily seen, regardless of whether they are surrounded by opacified or unopacified urine, although the lesions along the posterior aspect of the bladder are better seen on the wide window image. These abnormalities are also detected on an average intensity projection image obtained with intermediate (15 mm) thickness (D).

Diagnosis: Multifocal transitional cell carcinoma

Discussion: The differential diagnosis of multiple bladder masses includes both malignant and benign processes. Multifocal transitional cell carcinoma (TCC) is certainly a distinct possibility, although rarely severe chronic cystitis can have a similar appearance. Follow-up cystoscopy is warranted.

This case illustrates the frequent multifocal nature of bladder cancers at the time of detection. Thin section reformatted images have comparable sensitivity in detecting urinary tract pathology to axial images and provide an orientation often preferred by urologists. However, as with axial images, wide windowing (usually using windows of 2,000 to 4,000 HU and levels of 500 to 1,000 HU) is essential to maximize sensitivity in detecting small lesions located adjacent to densely opacified urine. Although three-dimensional reconstructions of thick slabs are insensitive in detecting bladder abnormalities (see Case 10-4), three-dimensional reconstructions of intermediate thickness have intermediate sensitivities. When the findings are extensive, as in this case, reconstructions of intermediate thickness (or less) will usually identify bladder masses.

History: 68-year-old male with persistent microscopic hematuria. History of prior, successfully treated, superficial bladder cancer and of transurethral resection of the prostate. Recent negative cystoscopy.

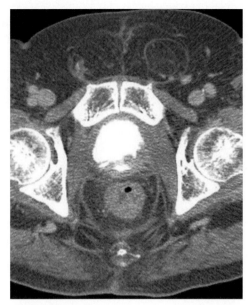

Figure 10.6   A

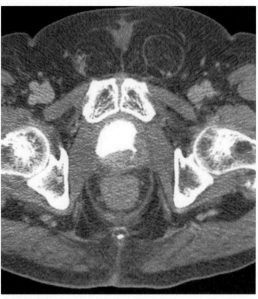

Figure 10.6   B

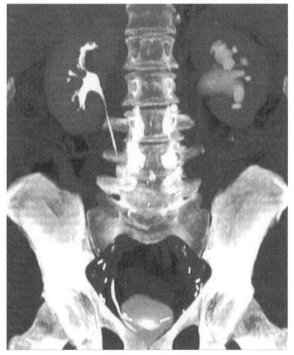

Figure 10.6   C

Findings: Two axial excretory phase CT urographic images (A, B) through the base of the bladder are provided. The urine in the bladder lumen is homogeneously opacified with excreted contrast material. A small amount of contrast material extends directly posteriorly in the midline, opacifying the defect from the transurethral resection of the prostate. There is asymmetric thickening of the left side of the bladder posteriorly. The interface between the bladder lumen and the bladder wall is slightly irregular. Bilateral inguinal hernias (containing only fat) are also incidentally noted. A maximum intensity projection coronal thick-slab image (C) does not demonstrate the bladder base abnormality.

Diagnosis: Transitional cell carcinoma

Discussion: It is difficult to differentiate prostatic enlargement from a bladder base wall abnormality, with the latter representing either focal changes of cystitis or, more likely, changes from a bladder neoplasm. Clues to the presence of a bladder wall abnormality include an irregular interface between the bladder lumen and wall and asymmetry in the appearance of the bladder lumen and bladder wall (both shown in this case).

Although cystoscopy is considered to be the gold standard for evaluation of the bladder for anatomic abnormalities, there are occasional false-negative cystoscopy results. This is more often true with cancers arising along the anterior wall of the bladder and at the bladder base. It is easy to understand why bladder base cancers may be missed at cystoscopy. Visualization of these neoplasms requires that the cystoscope be angled back upon itself. This may be particularly difficult in patients whose bladder bases are elevated by enlarged prostate glands.

History: 52-year-old female with one episode of gross hematuria.

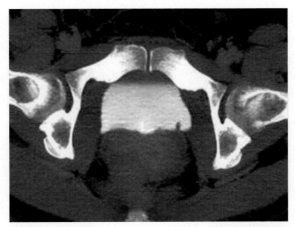

Figure 10.7   A

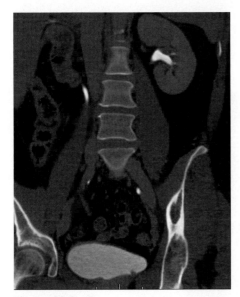

Figure 10.7   B

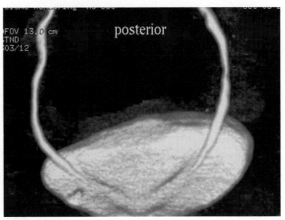

Figure 10.7   C

Findings: A single excretory phase axial CT urographic image filmed at wide windows (A) demonstrates a tiny 3 mm filling mass along the posterior aspect of the left side of the bladder. A thin section coronal image filmed at wide windows (B) also demonstrates the lesion, along the inferior aspect of the bladder, on the left. In addition, the lesion can also be identified on the posteroanterior volume-rendered image (C) as a small mass just caudal to the left ureterovesical junction. The mass could not be seen on the anteroposterior view.

Diagnosis: Tiny papillary transitional cell carcinoma

Discussion: As with excretory urography, the differential diagnosis for filling defects includes tumor, blood clot, and fungus ball; however, stone is unlikely because nearly all urinary tract calculi are of high CT attenuation (appearing similar to that of contrast-enhanced urine in the bladder lumen on excretory phase CT urographic images). By far the most likely diagnosis in a patient with a single tiny filling defect is urothelial neoplasm.

Tiny urothelial abnormalities can be detected with CT urography. In this instance, the detected lesion can be seen with multiple reconstruction techniques. Use of wide windowing is essential for all images, however, because the tiny lesion would be completely obscured by volume averaging with adjacent densely opacified urine if images were viewed using narrow windows.

Tiny papillary transitional cell carcinomas are often low grade and rarely invade the urothelium. Thus, they can usually be definitely treated (snared and removed) during cystoscopy.

History: Elderly man with hematuria.

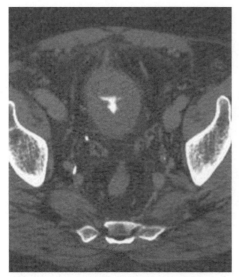

Figure 10.8   A

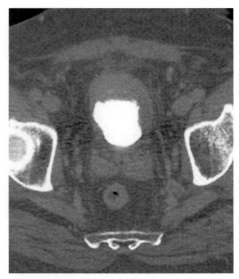

Figure 10.8   B

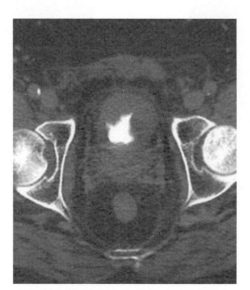

Figure 10.8   C

Findings: Three excretory phase axial images (A–C) from a CT urogram demonstrate marked diffuse bladder wall thickening. The bladder lumen is narrowed and the bladder wall surface irregular.

Diagnosis: Diffuse transitional cell carcinoma

Discussion: Diffuse bladder wall thickening is usually due to either muscular hypertrophy as a result of outlet obstruction, neurogenic bladders, or changes from cystitis. Rarely, bladder cancer can produce diffuse rather than focal wall thickening and can have an appearance indistinguishable from severe changes from the previously described benign entities. In such patients, history and physical examination may facilitate differentiation. Follow-up evaluation with cystoscopy is warranted.

History: 64-year-old male with positive urine cytology status post treatment of superficial bladder cancer.

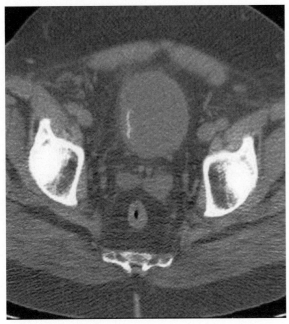

Figure 10.9   A

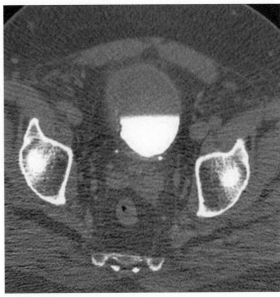

Figure 10.9   B

Findings: Two axial images from a CT urogram are provided. The first image (A), obtained prior to administration of contrast material, demonstrates a thin rim of linear calcification along the surface of a thickened right lateral wall of the bladder. The second image (B), obtained during the excretory phase after contrast material administration, confirms the presence of focal bladder wall thickening on the right and anteriorly.

Diagnosis: Scarring in right lateral bladder wall and missed cancer in left lateral bladder wall

Discussion: This case illustrates how CT urography can detect many anatomic abnormalities but often cannot distinguish between benign and malignant pathology. Thickening on the right was the result of scarring due to prior local treatment of the superficial bladder cancer. Linear calcification along the bladder wall at this location suggests that the changes were likely chronic and due to scarring. Calcification in bladder cancer is rare and, when present, is often more focal. This case also illustrates that some bladder cancers cannot be detected on CT urography. At cystoscopy, this patient was found to have a superficial cancer along the left lateral wall of the bladder. This neoplasm cannot be identified, even in retrospect. Although it is the opinion of many investigators that CT urography has improved sensitivity in detecting bladder cancers compared to both excretory urography and cystography, it cannot be used to detect all cancers, particularly those that are small or flat.

History: 57-year-old male with persistent microscopic hematuria.

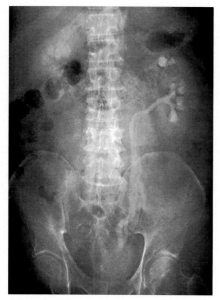

Figure 10.10   A

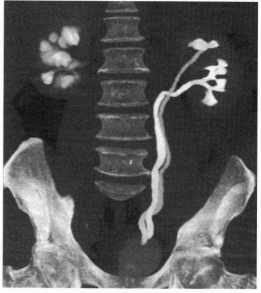

Figure 10.10   B

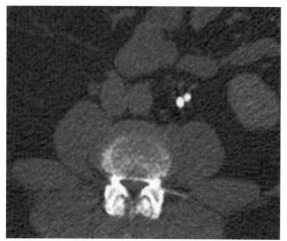

Figure 10.10   C

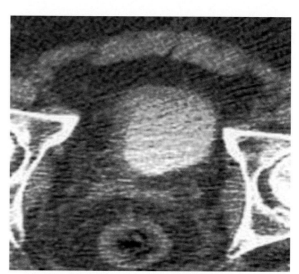

Figure 10.10   D

Findings: Excretory phase enhanced digital CT radiograph (A) and a thick-slab maximum intensity projection radiograph (B) obtained during a CT urogram demonstrate an asymmetric contour of the bladder. The bladder is displaced to the left, suggesting that there is a right-sided pelvic mass. The mass is obstructing the right renal collecting system since there is moderate to severe right hydronephrosis and the right ureter is not opacified. Finally, complete duplication of the left renal collecting system is also noted. Two excretory phase axial CT images are also provided. An image through the lower abdomen (C) demonstrates an unopacified mildly dilated right ureter and two opacified left ureters. Finally, an image through the mid pelvis (D) reveals the distorted contour of the bladder. Although the enhanced scout and the maximum intensity projection image suggest otherwise, these images indicate that the abnormal appearance of the bladder is due to focal right lateral wall thickening, the most common cause of which is urothelial neoplasm.

Diagnosis: Transitional cell carcinoma obstructing the right renal collecting system

Discussion: This case illustrates that conventional radiography (as illustrated by the enhanced digital CT radiograph) and three-dimensional images may be misleading in identifying the etiology of a bladder abnormality because these techniques only image the bladder lumen rather than the bladder wall. In comparison, nonobstructed duplicated renal collecting systems are easily identified on both axial and coronal images.

History: 52-year-old male with positive urine cytology status post treatment of superficial bladder cancers.

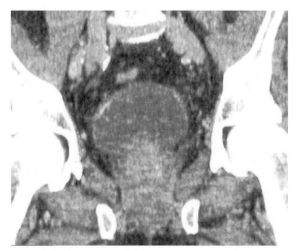

Figure 10.11   A

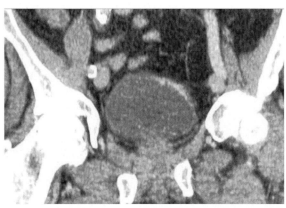

Figure 10.11   B

Findings: Two thin section coronal nephrographic phase images through the pelvis (A, B) show that the bladder wall is thickened diffusely. However, there are two focal linear areas of increased attenuation at the dome of the bladder—one on the right (A) and one on the left (B). In addition, an enlarged prostate gland impresses upon and elevates the bladder base.

Diagnosis: Two flat transitional cell carcinomas at the dome of the bladder and benign prostatic hyperplasia

Discussion: Bladder cancers often demonstrate brisk hyperenhancement after administration of contrast material, relative to the normal less intensely enhancing bladder wall. In this case, two bladder neoplasms can be identified primarily due to their hyperenhancement. Hyperenhancement is often best seen on nephrographic phase images (if they are extended through the pelvis) but can also be detected on excretory phase scans. Although nephrographic phase images can facilitate identification of some urothelial neoplasms, such as the case illustrated here, their routine use through the pelvis is not warranted (unless they are obtained in combination with excretory phase scans with a split bolus contrast material injection). It is desirable to limit patient radiation exposure. When the split bolus technique is employed, however, the bladder lumen is usually at least partially opacified with excreted contrast material. This may make it more difficult to identify flat enhancing tumors in the bladder wall. Fortunately, in most patients, neoplasms can be detected on excretory phase images primarily because they are well outlined by the opacified high-attenuation or unopacified water attenuation urine in the adjacent bladder lumen.

History: 47-year-old female with recurrent urinary tract infections with mild cystitis diagnosed at cystoscopy.

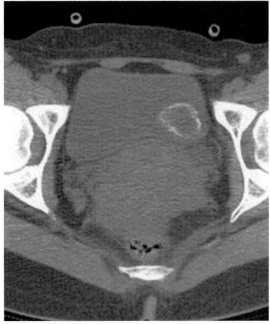

Figure 10.12   A

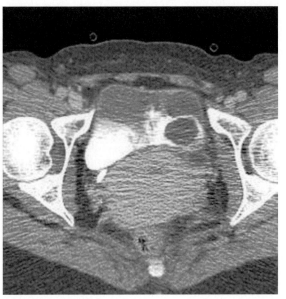

Figure 10.12   B

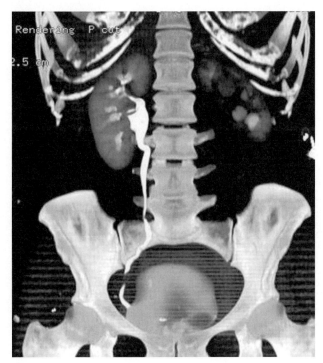

Figure 10.12   C

Findings: An unenhanced axial image (A) demonstrates an ovoid ring-shaped calcification in the left posterolateral aspect of the bladder. An excretory phase axial image (B) demonstrates a smoothly marginated ovoid mass along the left posterolateral aspect of the bladder. The volume-rendered image (C) shows the ovoid mass in the left infero-lateral aspect of the bladder, appearing as a filling defect. The left side of the urinary tract is obstructed, resulting in left pelvocaliectasis and an unopacified left ureter.

Diagnosis: Leiomyoma

Discussion: Benign bladder tumors are rare, with the most common benign tumor being a leiomyoma. Bladder leiomyomas most frequently occur near the trigone, as in this case. Calcification has been reported infrequently. The overlying mucosa is almost always intact. For this reason, cystoscopy may be normal or may demonstrate only mild or moderate deformity of the intact overlying urothelium. Patients rarely present with hematuria. The diagnosis of leiomyoma can be suspected on imaging studies when a smoothly marginated bladder mass is identified and makes a characteristic right angle with the bladder wall, suggesting that it is intra-mural in location. Confirmation with cystoscopy is always required since these tumors cannot be definitively distin-guished from bladder malignancies.

Possible diagnostic considerations in this case would include an unusual bladder neoplasm (given the rim of peripheral calcification), laminated calculus, or calcifica-tion within a chronic blood clot or fungus ball. The first two possibilities are most likely.

History: 51-year-old male with recurrent urinary tract infections.

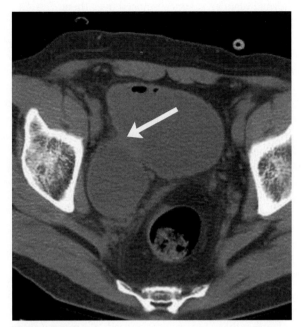

Figure 10.13   A

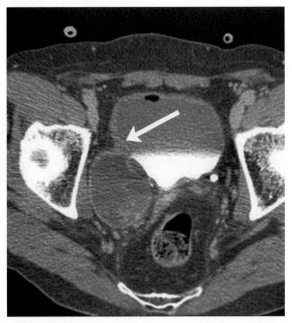

Figure 10.13   B

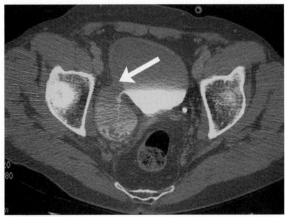

Figure 10.13   C

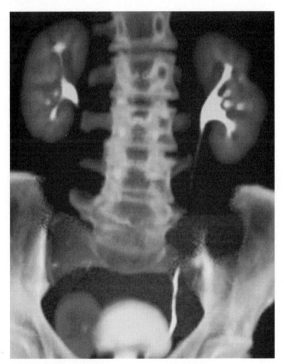

Figure 10.13   D

Findings: An unenhanced image of the pelvis (A) shows a water attenuation mass along the right posterior aspect of the bladder. This could represent either a bladder diverticulum or a cystic mass separate from the bladder. Two axial excretory phase images through the bladder, one obtained at 300 seconds (B) and the other at 450 seconds (C), demonstrate that the large mass projects from the right posterolateral aspect of the bladder. Excreted contrast material layers dependently in this structure and multiple small filling defects are present (C). In addition, mild wall thickening (arrows) is seen in the neck of the diverticulum (A–C). A volume-rendered image (D) also demonstrates the faintly opacified collection of urine in the right hemipelvis, as well as a collection of contrast material in the prostatic fossa.

Diagnosis: Large bladder diverticulum, containing a small urothelial neoplasm in its neck, in a patient who has had a prior transurethral resection of the prostate

Discussion: Bladder diverticula are acquired abnormalities in the vast majority of instances, usually forming as a result of bladder outlet obstruction or a neurogenic bladder. Only rarely are they congenital. Acquired bladder diverticula are false diverticula because they represent herniations of bladder mucosa through submucosa. These may occasionally be difficult to detect on anteroposterior radiographs obtained during excretory urography or cystography because the majority of bladder diverticula extend posteriorly, such that the normal bladder is superimposed over them.

There are a number of complications of bladder diverticula. Urine may accumulate within acquired diverticula during voiding and result in the desire to urinate again immediately after initial voiding is complete. Bladder diverticula can also serve as a cause of urinary stasis, resulting in an increased likelihood of urinary tract infections. Bladder calculi may also form. Finally, bladder neoplasms may develop, as in this case. When this happens, the neoplasms may be aggressive because they are not contained by submucosal, muscular, or serosal layers. In this patient, the bladder wall thickening at the neck of the diverticulum was demonstrated at cystoscopy to represent a transitional cell carcinoma.

Neoplasms in bladder diverticula may demonstrate a variety of imaging appearances: focal diverticular wall thickening (as illustrated here), a mural filling detect, or diffuse wall thickening. In rare instances, the diverticulum may be completely filled with soft tissue. The multiple tiny filling defects located at the base of the diverticulum in this case were subsequently determined to represent small blood clots.

CASE 10-14

History: 84-year-old male with urinary frequency.

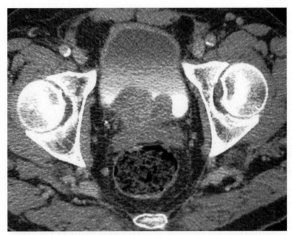

Figure 10.14 A

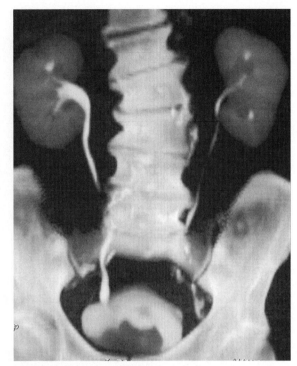

Figure 10.14 B

Findings: An excretory phase axial image (A) demonstrates a large lobulated mass projecting into the bladder lumen from the posterior wall. On the volume-rendered image (B), the mass can also be seen to extend into the bladder lumen from the bladder base.

Diagnosis: Marked benign prostatic hyperplasia

Discussion: In an elderly male, the most common mass located at the bladder base and projecting into the bladder lumen is an enlarged prostate gland. This is almost always due to benign prostatic hyperplasia. In this patient, the mass could be seen on other images to be contiguous with the more inferior components of the prostate gland. Although cancer of the bladder base could invade the prostate gland and have a similar appearance, this is a much less likely possibility. Cystoscopy is recommended in patients with this finding.

History: 45-year-old female with recurrent urinary tract infections.

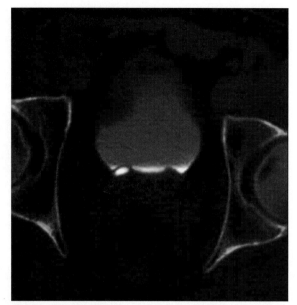

Figure 10.15   A

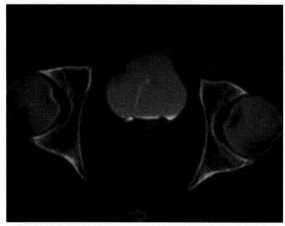

Figure 10.15   B

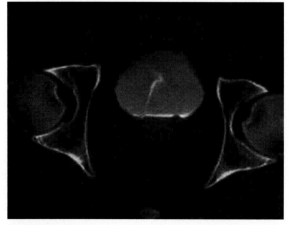

Figure 10.15   C

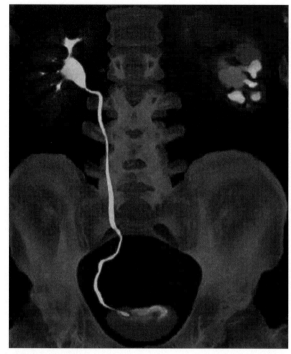

Figure 10.15   D

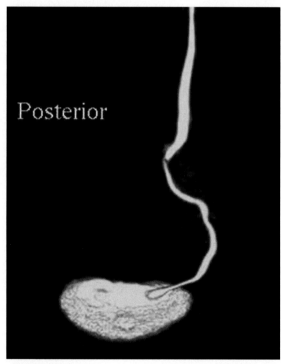

Figure 10.15   E

Findings: Three excretory phase axial images (A–C) demonstrate the right ureter inserting into the bladder. On the two more cephalad images (A, B), the distal-most right ureter is prominent and there is a uniform thin rim of soft tissue along its anterior and medial aspects (between the ureter and opacified urine in the bladder lumen). On the most caudal image (C), a jet of opacified urine projects into the bladder lumen, which contains inhomogeneously mixed contrast material-containing and unenhanced urine. The abnormality of the distal right ureter is more easily characterized on the anteroposterior (D) maximum intensity projection images and on the posteroanterior volume-rendered image (E), on which the smooth distal dilatation is again identified, along with the surrounding uniform thin rim of soft tissue.

Diagnosis: Small orthotopic (simple) ureterocele

Discussion: Small ureteroceles can be detected with CT urography, but their appearance may be subtle on axial images. In these cases, the ureteroceles may be easier to identify on coronal or coronal oblique images (see Case 4-12).

Orthotopic or simple ureteroceles are often incidental findings in patients without duplicating renal collecting systems, and they are frequently asymptomatic. In comparison, ectopic ureteroceles are found in patients with duplicated renal collecting systems. These ureteroceles usually involve the ureter draining the upper pole moiety because it inserts abnormally into the bladder inferior and medial to the normal upper pole moiety ureteral insertion site. Ectopic ureteroceles may obstruct the renal collecting system and ureter (see Case 9-23). When large, ureteroceles may produce filling defects in the bladder that can mimic neoplasms on excretory urography, although distinction is usually easily made with CT urography.

History: Elderly man previously treated for prostate cancer with urinary frequency.

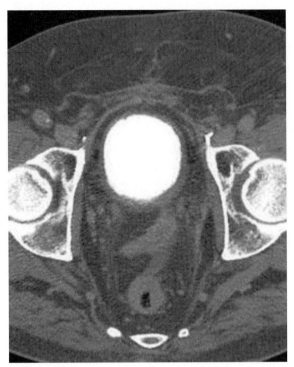

Figure 10.16

Findings: A single excretory phase axial CT image demonstrates mild diffuse circumferential bladder wall thickening, which is slightly more pronounced along the posterior aspect of the bladder. There are no filling defects in the bladder lumen. There is increased soft tissue attenuation and linear stranding in the adjacent perivesical fat.

Diagnosis: Radiation cystitis

Discussion: Bladder wall thickening is caused by both benign and malignant diseases of the bladder; however, the distribution of thickening usually suggests which type of disease is present. In most cases, diffuse bladder wall thickening is the result of cystitis, regardless of cause, or related to muscular hypertrophy from bladder outlet obstruction or neurogenic bladder. In comparison, most bladder cancers produce focal bladder wall thickening. Only in rare instances do some infiltrative bladder cancers produce diffuse bladder wall thickening; in these cases, there is usually some asymmetry to the pattern of thickening. Cystitis only rarely results in focal bladder wall thickening.

There are many causes of chronic cystitis, each of which can lead to bladder wall thickening and diminished bladder compliance and/or capacity. These include hemorrhagic cystitis (usually from cyclophosphamide therapy), radiation cystitis (as in this case), and infection (which may be due to chronic bacterial infection, schistosomiasis, or tuberculosis). Other inflammatory conditions, including cystitis glandularis, malakoplakia, and cystitis cystica, may also be responsible for bladder wall thickening. Distinction of the cause of cystitis is frequently not possible, although calcification is more common with schistosomiasis.

Cystitis may result from external beam radiation therapy, either immediately or as a delayed response. This most commonly occurs when radiation is administered to patients with cervical, prostate, or bladder cancer and when the radiation dose exceeds 40 Gy. The acute phase of radiation cystitis results in active inflammation and edema, whereas the chronic phase (developing between 1 and 4 years after treatment) results in vasculitis and fibrosis. The bladder capacity is usually reduced in patients with chronic radiation cystitis. Patients often have persistent hematuria.

In many cases, patients with acute cystitis will not have any CT urography-detectable abnormalities; however, when there is severe bladder involvement, extensive wall thickening may be encountered. In comparison, CT urography-detectable abnormalities are frequently identified in patients with chronic cystitis.

CASE 10-17

History: 45-year-old male with intractable urinary tract infections.

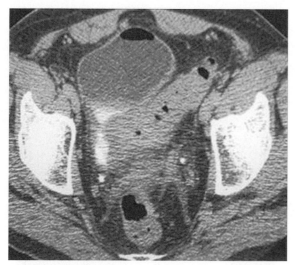

Figure 10.17   A

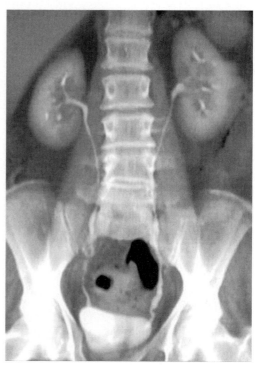

Figure 10.17   B

Findings: An excretory phase axial CT urographic image (A) demonstrates nondependent air in the bladder lumen. The bladder wall is smoothly thickened. In addition, the interface between the bladder and the adjacent sigmoid colon is obscured and the colon is thick walled. A single coronal average intensity projection image (B) does not show the intraluminal bladder air or the bladder wall thickening, and the sigmoid colon cannot be visualized.

Diagnosis: Colovesical fistula secondary to diverticulitis

Discussion: The peak age for developing a fistula between the bladder and bowel is the mid-fifties to mid-sixties. Fistulae are more commonly encountered in men. Although there are a number of diseases that can produce fistulae between the bladder and adjacent bowel, the most common cause of a colovesical fistula is diverticulitis. It has been estimated that such fistulae occur in 2% of patients with diverticulitis. Symptoms from a colovesical fistula are initially nonspecific, usually related to the presence of cystitis,

which does not resolve with treatment. More specific symptoms of pneumaturia or fecaluria do not develop until later.

CT is the most sensitive study for detecting bladder fistulae, primarily because of its ability to detect even small amounts of air in the bladder lumen (seen in 90% or more of cases). Because the diagnosis is frequently dependent on the ability to detect air in the bladder lumen, it is imperative that the patient not be instrumented within 24 hours of the CT scan. In this way, any air that is present can be identified definitively as pathologic rather than iatrogenic. Often, the adjacent involved bowel will be thick-walled. The fistula is commonly not identified. In comparison, cystography and even cystoscopy are able to identify fistulae from bladder to colon in fewer than half of patients.

In this case, the diagnosis of vesicocolic fistula can be made only on the axial CT images. This is another example in which the three-dimensionally reconstructed images are not helpful.

History: 51- (A, B) and 72-year-old (C, D) males status post surgery for bladder cancer.

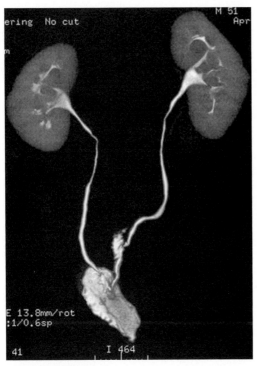

Figure 10.18   A

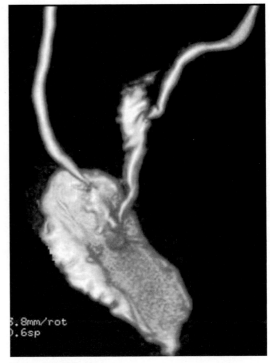

Figure 10.18   B

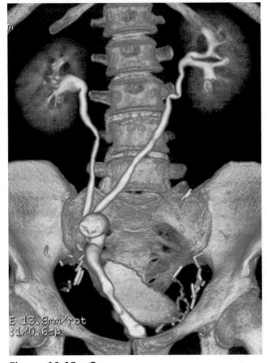

Figure 10.18   C

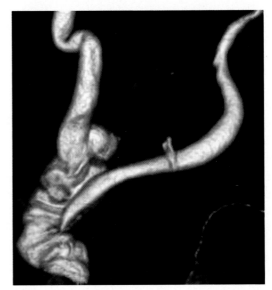

Figure 10.18   D

Findings: Volume-rendered images are provided for two different patients [(A and B) for 51-year-old, and (C and D) for 72 year-old]. Anteroposterior and coned-down oblique views are provided for each patient. In both patients, both ureters are noted to anastomose to loops of ileum, which then extend down toward the bladder fossae, where larger urinary reservoirs are identified.

Diagnosis: Normal postoperative anatomy after cystectomy and creation of an ileal neobladder

Discussion: Three different basic types of urinary diversions are used. The simplest is the ileal loop diversion, in which the ureters are anastomosed to a loop of ileum, which is then brought out to the anterior abdominal wall at an ostomy. These diversions are refluxing and the patients are incontinent. The patient wears an ostomy bag that collects excreted urine. A more recently developed approach has been the creation of continent reservoirs made of ileum, colon, or both (e.g., Kock and Indiana pouches). These reservoirs are also connected to the anterior abdominal wall at an ostomy. Urine does not drain spontaneously from the reservoir to the anterior abdominal wall because the reservoir is connected in such a fashion (via intussusception of its limbs)

as to prevent both reflux into the ureters and incontinence. Patients are required to catheterize the reservoir regularly throughout the day, usually every 4 to 8 hours. Most recently, creation of an orthotopic neobladder, from ileum, has been performed. This procedure is highly desirable because the newly created urinary reservoir is directly anastomosed to the urethra, and many patients are continent. There is no requirement for an ostomy bag or for intermittent catheterization of the reservoir. In most patients, both ureters are anastomosed to an "afferent limb" of ileum that is usually placed anteriorly and then connected to a larger reservoir constructed from a cross-folded loop of ileum, which sits in the bladder fossa. This second segment of ileum is then anastomosed to the urethra.

CT urography can be used to demonstrate postoperative anatomy and evaluate patients after cystectomy and urinary diversion. Of particular note is the ability of CT urography to demonstrate the uretero-ileal anastomoses, as shown in the cases illustrated here. Three-dimensional reconstructions are particularly helpful; however, all anatomic information is displayed on the source axial images.

History: 64-year-old male with fever following radical cystectomy.

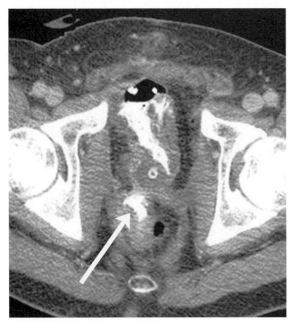

Figure 10.19   A

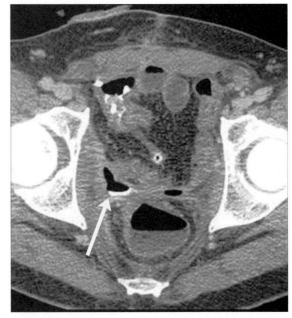

Figure 10.19   B

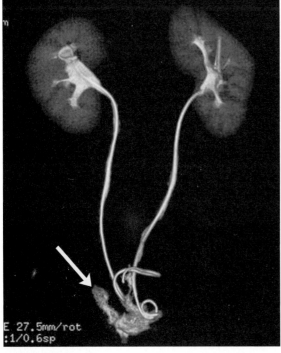

Figure 10.19   C

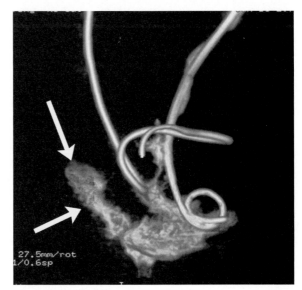

Figure 10.19   D

Findings: An axial excretory phase image (A) demonstrates excreted contrast material and air in the bladder, with the bladder also containing a fluid-filled balloon of a Foley catheter. A small collection of contrast material just posterolateral to the Foley balloon lies outside of the bladder (arrow). A slightly more cephalad axial image (B) also reveals air and contrast material in the extraperitoneal collection along the right pelvic sidewall (arrow). The size and orientation of the collection are also seen on two volume-rendered images (arrows), the first an anteroposterior image including both renal collecting systems and ureters (C) and the second a coned-down right posterior oblique image (D). The three-dimensional images also demonstrate the presence of indwelling stents in both ureters (although they are partially obscured by contrast material in the ureters).

Diagnosis: Leak from anastomosis of ileal neobladder to urethra

Discussion: Urine may leak from the anastomosis of the ileal neobladder to the urethra after cystectomy. In this case, the size and location of the leak (including its origin from the base of the reservoir) are demonstrated on the axial images but are easier to visualize on the three-dimensional images. This extraluminal collection can be distinguished from the afferent limb due to its posterolateral location and its amorphous shape.

CT urography can also be used effectively to evaluate patients for other complications after urinary diversion. In a review by Sudakoff and associates, CT urography was performed to assess 24 patients with urinary diversions for tumor recurrence or diversion malfunction. Nine abnormalities, including strictures in four patients, urinary tract dilatation, calculus formation in the reservoir, and recurrent tumor, were detected.

This patient was treated successfully with prolonged upper tract decompression and Foley catheter placement. If the leak had not healed, the patient would have had to return to the operating room for open surgical repair.

History: 72-year-old male with hematuria following cystectomy and creation of an ileal neobladder for bladder cancer.

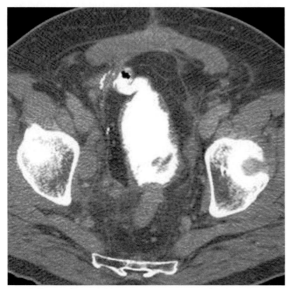

Figure 10.20   A

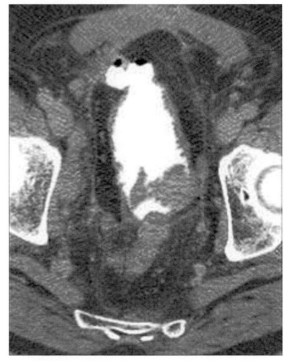

Figure 10.20   B

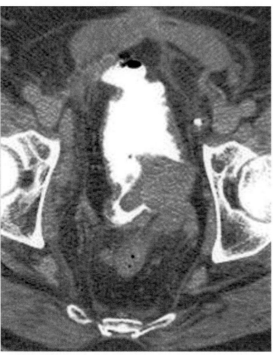

Figure 10.20   C

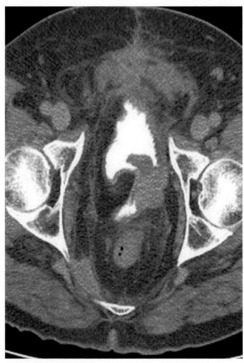

Figure 10.20   D

Findings: Four excretory phase axial images from a CT urogram are provided (A–D), extending from the cephalic aspect of the ileal reservoir (A) to the caudal aspect (D). The images demonstrate a large amount of excreted contrast material within the neobladder, some of which surrounds a large soft tissue mass located on the left posteriorly.

Diagnosis: Recurrent transitional cell carcinoma in left hemipelvis involving the left lateral aspect of the neobladder

Discussion: Transitional cell carcinomas can recur locally following cystectomy. In one series, local recurrences were identified in 12% of patients, with a median time to recurrence of 10 months. In most instances, recurrences result in the development of tumor masses or enlarged lymph nodes in the pelvis, some of which can grow to be quite large. It is unusual for recurrences to involve the neobladder directly. In a series reported by Hautmann and Simon, only 10 of 43 recurrences in patients with neobladders involved the neobladder (producing obstruction or malignant infiltration, as in this case). Some, but not all, patients with local recurrences in the pelvis also have distant metastatic disease. Patients with a history of bladder cancer are also at increased risk for developing upper urinary tract neoplasms.

Ileal neobladders often have a lobulated shape and their walls usually appear slightly thickened. However, a normal neobladder does not contain as much soft tissue as in this case. Recurrent tumor should be considered.

History: 67-year-old male with hematuria.

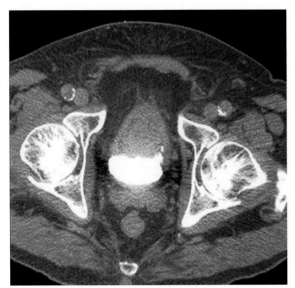

Figure 10.21   A

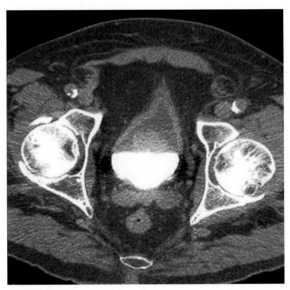

Figure 10.21   B

Findings: Two excretory phase axial images (A, B) through the bladder demonstrate layering of unenhanced urine anterior to denser contrast-containing urine in the bladder lumen. The bladder wall is circumferentially thickened. In addition, there is a 4-cm round soft tissue attenuation mass projecting into the bladder lumen along its anterior and lateral portions, where it is outlined by opacified or minimally opacified urine in the bladder lumen. There is no abnormal perivesical stranding, and no enlarged pelvic lymph nodes are identified.

Diagnosis: Transitional cell carcinoma

Discussion: Occasionally, large bladder cancers may be difficult to identify with CT urography, particularly when these neoplasms lie primarily or entirely within portions of the bladder that do not contain opacified urine. In these instances, the likelihood of detection is increased if images are viewed using narrow windows (to maximize the density differences between the soft tissue attenuation tumor and water attenuation unenhanced urine). This case illustrates that although wide window viewing is necessary to maximize sensitivity in detecting lesions within or adjacent to contrast-containing urine, soft tissue window viewing is also sometimes required.

The problem of unopacified urine can usually be avoided by having patients void just prior to their exams. Another possible solution is to ask the patient to ambulate for several minutes and then roll over on the CT table several times before excretory phase imaging is performed. These maneuvers facilitate homogeneous mixing of contrast material and urine in the bladder, effectively eliminating the problem encountered in this case. We do not perform this last maneuver routinely because it adds complexity to the CT scan. Patients who ambulate must be carefully repositioned on the CT table after they have exercised. Also, it is our belief that, as this case shows, as long as images through the bladder are carefully reviewed and narrow windowing is utilized, the probability of missing a bladder cancer is low.

History: 43-year-old female with multiple urinary tract infections.

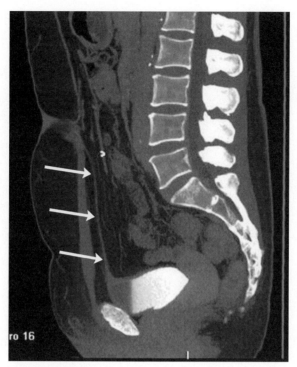

Figure 10.22

Findings: A single sagittal image at the midline of the lower abdomen and pelvis demonstrates dependently layering contrast material in the bladder. The anterior portion of the bladder contains unopacified urine. There is a linear projection of soft tissue (arrows) extending superiorly and anteriorly from the dome of the bladder to the umbilicus.

Diagnosis: Urachal remnant

Discussion: The urachus forms as an embryologic diverticulum that grows anteriorly and cranially from the cloaca. Initially, the urachus represents a way by which the bladder extends all the way to the anterior abdominal wall at the umbilicus. Functionally, the urachus closes prior to birth in the vast majority of patients. After birth, the closed urachal remnant may still be visualized and is termed the median umbilical ligament. In this patient, the urachus does not contain fluid and does not appear to communicate with the bladder. Similarly, on physical examination, there was no apparent communication with the umbilicus.

There are four urachal anomalies that may develop and that can produce symptoms: a patent urachus (which communicates with both the bladder and the umbilicus), a urachal cyst (which does not directly communicate with the bladder or umbilicus), a urachal sinus (which communicates only with the umbilicus), and a urachal diverticulum (which communicates only with the bladder). Urachal cysts may occasionally become infected. Another important complication of urachal remnants is carcinoma, which, unlike bladder cancers, is usually adenocarcinoma rather than transitional cell carcinoma.

CT urography can be used to detect all types of urachal remnants, including the asymptomatic median umbilical ligament. Unlike intravenous urography or cystography, or even a sinus tract injection, detection does not rely on the demonstration of contrast material within the urachal remnant.

History: 88-year-old female with persistent gross hematuria.

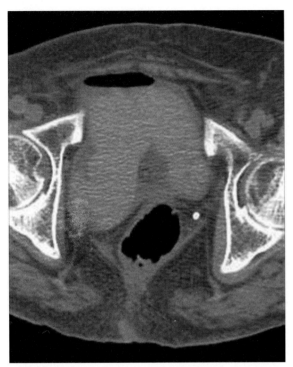

Figure 10.23 A

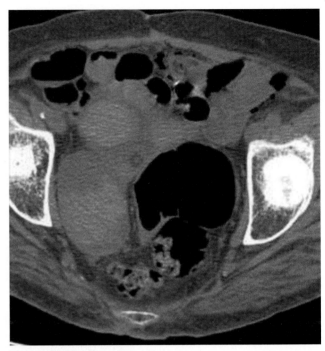

Figure 10.23 B

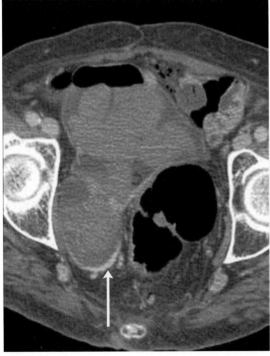

Figure 10.23 C

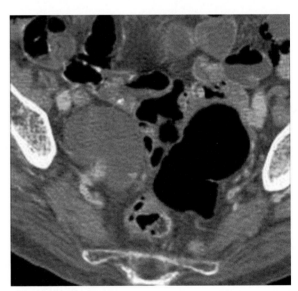

Figure 10.23 D

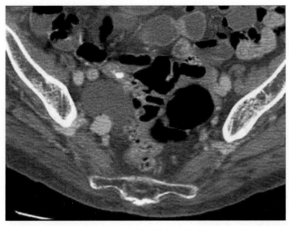

Figure 10.23   E

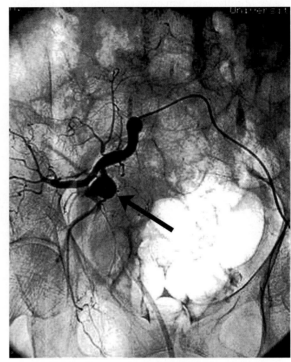

Figure 10.23   F

Findings: Two unenhanced axial images from a CT uro-gram are provided. The first (A) demonstrates a large amount of high-attenuation material in the bladder. The high-attenuation material also extends into a diverticulum extending from the right posterolateral aspect of the bladder, as seen on the second image (B). Air in the bladder lumen is from a recent catheterization. Nephrographic phase images through the pelvis reveal the same high-attenuation mater-ial in the bladder lumen as well as in the right-sided diverticulum; however, there is a small amount of high-attenuation material (arrow) layering posteriorly in the diverticulum (C). A slightly more cephalic image (D) shows that this high-attenuation material is immediately contigu-ous to an enhancing vessel, which is aneurysmally dilated on the final axial image (E). A subsequent image from an arteriogram (F), obtained after selective injection of the right internal iliac artery, demonstrates that the dilated structure seen on the CT urogram is a focal aneurysm of the right internal iliac artery (arrow).

Diagnosis: Arteriovesical fistula from right internal iliac artery aneurysm to bladder diverticulum

Discussion: Fistulae between the bladder and adjacent bowel or the vagina are fairly common. In contrast, com-munications between pelvic arteries and the bladder are exceedingly rare, with only a few cases reported in the liter-ature. When fistulae are present, they may occur between the bladder and the common iliac, internal iliac, or external iliac arteries. Several different etiologies have been identi-fied: pelvic trauma (pseudoaneurysm formation and rupture after a gunshot wound); iatrogenic injuries following renal and/or pancreatic transplantation; and vascular disease such as atherosclerosis, in which case the patient should have evi-dence of aneurysmal disease in other vessels. Arteriovesical fistulae should be considered in the differential diagnosis in patients with any of these diseases who have persistent or recurrent unexplained hematuria.

In this patient, the availability of nephrographic phase images through the pelvis greatly facilitated the diagnosis by demonstrating active extravasation of contrast material from the internal iliac artery into a bladder diverticulum. Although nephrographic phase images are not routinely obtained through the pelvis, these images (or images obtained even sooner after the contrast material injection begins) can occasionally be useful in patients for whom there is concern about the integrity of the pelvic vasculature.

It is possible that the development of a fistula in this patient was made easier due to the fact that it occurred between the iliac artery and a bladder diverticulum. Since the majority of bladder diverticula are pseudodiverticula, repre-senting acquired herniations of bladder mucosa through the submucosa, most bladder diverticula are not surrounded by all layers of the bladder wall.

History: Middle-aged female with pelvic pain and hematuria.

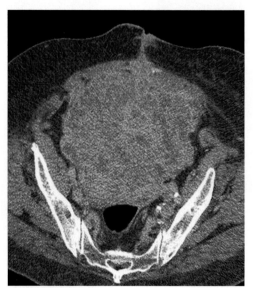

Figure 10.24 A

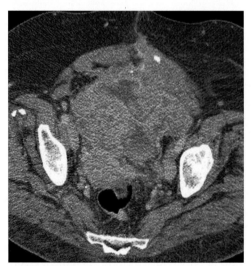

Figure 10.24 B

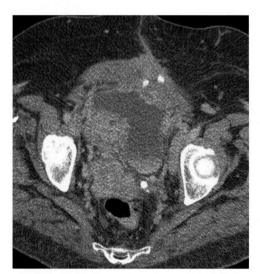

Figure 10.24 C

Findings: Three excretory phase axial CT images (A–C) demonstrate a large heterogeneous pelvic mass, with its center cephalad to the bladder. The mass extends into the right lateral aspect of the bladder and deforms the bladder lumen.

Diagnosis: Uterine leiomyosarcoma with bladder invasion

Discussion: Rarely, extrinsic malignant processes may extend to and invade through the bladder wall. These are usually due to malignancies in contiguous organs, such as the prostate gland, seminal vesicles, uterus, cervix, or vagina. Microscopic invasion will not be detected on CT urography; however, gross invasion, as is present in this patient, is usually identified. A uterine origin can be suspected in this patient, given the location of the center of the mass. Although uterine fibroids are often heterogeneous, they rarely produce such a large amount of irregularly enhancing soft tissue. For this reason, malignancy should be considered.

CASE 10-25

History: Middle-aged patient with gross hematuria.

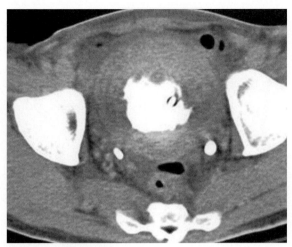

Figure 10.25   A

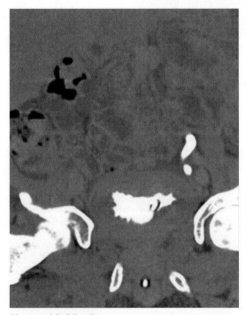

Figure 10.25   B

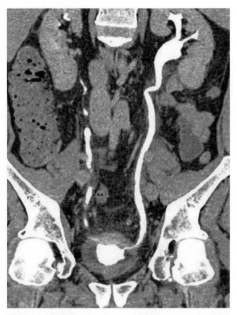

Figure 10.25   C

Findings: Axial (A) and coronal (B) images through the bladder demonstrate severe diffuse, circumferential bladder wall thickening, with the bladder wall thickness exceeding 1 cm.

Diagnosis: Hemorrhagic cystitis secondary to cyclophosphamide therapy

Discussion: This case illustrates a severe bladder abnormality. In general, severe diffuse bladder wall thickening is usually the result of muscular (detrusor) hypertrophy (related to bladder outlet obstruction or a neurogenic bladder) or to severe cystitis, although the differential diagnosis also includes diffuse bladder cancer and bladder involvement with lymphoma. A coronal CT urography image of another patient with detrusor hypertrophy (C) is also provided in

order to demonstrate the very similar appearances of different causes of severe diffuse bladder wall thickening. In patients with this degree of wall thickening, correlation with clinical history is often helpful. In this case, the patient had received chemotherapy for treatment of lymphoma.

Up to 40% of patients treated with cyclophosphamide can develop an acute cystitis; however, often the cystitis usually resolves without severe adverse sequelae. In some patients, hemorrhage may be severe and require angiographic embolization or cystectomy. In rare instances, bladder wall calcification will eventually develop. Patients who have received cyclophosphamide have an increased incidence of urinary tract cancer, especially bladder cancer. (Case courtesy of Stuart G. Silverman, MD, Brigham and Women's Hospital, Boston, MA.)

History: 53-year-old female with abdominal pain.

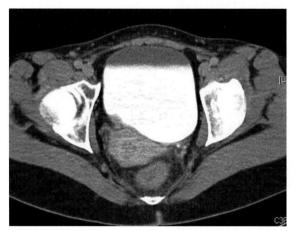

Figure 10.26   A

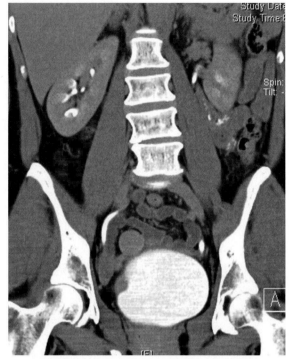

Figure 10.26   B

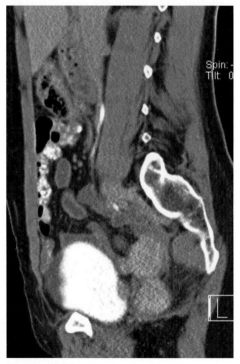

Figure 10.26   C

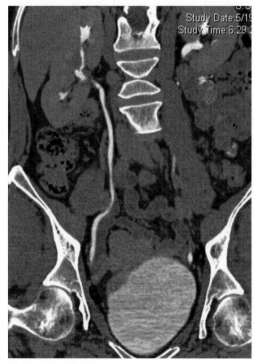

Figure 10.26   D

Findings: Axial CT image (A) demonstrates a small nodular mass along the right posterolateral aspect of the bladder lumen. The mass is also seen on coronal and sagittal reformatted images [(B and C), respectively] as well as on a curved multiplanar reformatted image (D). The bladder wall is not thickened elsewhere, and there are no filling defects noted in the bladder lumen. Finally, lobulated masses noted posterior to the bladder are associated with the uterus.

Diagnosis: Endometriosis of the bladder wall

Discussion: Endometriosis rarely affects the bladder. When it does, only the serosa of the bladder may be affected or a mural mass may project into and invade the bladder lumen, in which case patients will present with cyclical hematuria. On CT urography, the appearance is nonspecific. This small endometrioma is indistinguishable from a bladder neoplasm. This patient had a history of a previously cystoscopically resected endometrioma and had recurrent pain but no hematuria. On repeat cystoscopy, the urothelium was intact. Only an extrinsic impression was identified. This endometrioma had not invaded through the bladder wall. (Case courtesy of Stuart G. Silverman, MD, Brigham and Women's Hospital, Boston, MA.)

History: 55-year-old female with urinary tract infections and incontinence.

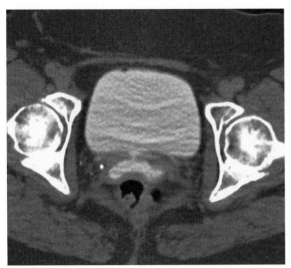

Figure 10.27 A

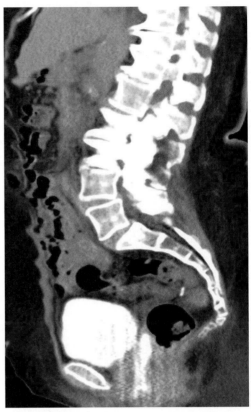

Figure 10.27 B

Findings: An axial excretory phase image (A) demonstrates a punctate collection of air in the anterior aspect of the bladder. Contrast-containing urine homogeneously opacifies the entire bladder. There is a smaller collection of contrast-enhanced urine located posterior to the bladder that appears to communicate with the bladder via a thin linear tract. The fistula from the bladder and the more posterior structure with which the fistula communicates are better seen on the sagittal reformatted image (B).

Diagnosis: Vesicovaginal fistula

Discussion: Vesicovaginal fistulae are most often encountered after gynecologic surgery. Usually, they are seen after hysterectomies have been performed for benign disease; however, they can also be seen in patients who have been treated for cervical carcinoma (usually with both surgery and radiation). Most patients with vesicovaginal fistulae present with continuous incontinence, although some will complain merely of a vaginal discharge. Although cystography or vaginography may demonstrate vesicovaginal fistulae, they can also be detected and specifically diagnosed with CT urography when intravenously administered excreted contrast material accumulates in the vagina on delayed images. (Case courtesy of Stuart G. Silverman, MD, Brigham and Women's Hospital, Boston, MA.)

SUGGESTED READINGS

1. Caoili EM, Cohan RH, Korobkin M, et al. Urinary tract abnormalities: initial experience with multi-detector row CT urography. *Radiology*. 2002;222:353–360.

2. Dunnick NR, Sandler CM, Newhouse JH, et al. *Textbook of uroradiology*. Philadelphia: Lippincott Williams & Wilkins; 2001.

3. Friedland GW, DeVries PA, Nino-Murcia M. Congenital anomalies of the urachus and bladder. In: Pollack HM, McLennan BL, Dyer R, et al., eds. *Clinical urography*. Philadelphia: Saunders; 2000:826–831.

4. Goff CD, Davidson JT, Teague N, et al. Hematuria from arteriovesical fistula: unusual presentation of ruptured iliac artery aneurysm. *Am Surg*. 1999;65:421–422.

5. Hautmann RE, Simon J. Ileal neobladder and local recurrence of bladder cancer: patterns of failure and impact on function in men. *J Urol*. 2000;164:128–129.

6. Jafri SZH, Roberts JL, Berger BD. Fistulas of the genitourinary tract. In: Pollack HM, McLennan BL, Dyer R, et al., eds. *Clinical urography*. Philadelphia: Saunders; 2000:3004–3006.

7. Kulkarni JN, Pramesh CS, Rathi S, et al. Long term results of orthotopic neobladder reconstruction after radical cystectomy. *BJU Int*. 2003;92:485–488.

8. Noroozian M, Cohan RH, Caoili EM, et al. Multislice CT urography: state of the art. *Br J Radiol*. 2004;77:S74–S86.

9. Patel U, Rickards D. *Imaging and urodynamics of the lower urinary tract*. Abington, UK: Taylor & Francis; 2005.

10. Saluja S, Lazzarini KM, Smith RC. Inflammation of the urinary bladder. In: Pollack HM, McLennan BL, Dyer R, et al., eds. *Clinical urography*. Philadelphia: Saunders; 2000:1033–1035.

11. Shah O, Ficazzola M, Torre P, et al. Arteriovesical fistula: a complication of bladder trauma. *J Urol*. 2001;166:996.

12. Spring DB, Deshon GE. Radiology of vesical and supravesical urinary diversions and orthotopic bladder replacements. In: Pollack HM, McLennan BL, Dyer R, et al., eds. *Clinical urography*. Philadelphia: Saunders; 2000:357–377.

13. Sudakoff GS, Guralnick M, Langenstroer P, et al. CT urography of urinary diversions with enhanced CT digital radiography: preliminary experience. *Am J Roentgenol*. 2005;184:131–138.

CHAPTER ELEVEN

CT UROGRAPHY PITFALLS AND ARTIFACTS

RICHARD H. COHAN, MD

ELAINE M. CAOILI, MD

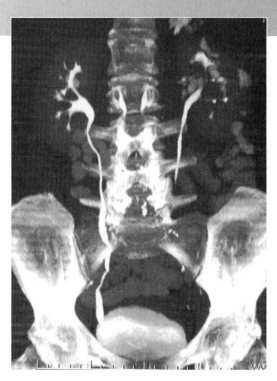

History: 55-year-old woman with intermittent hematuria.

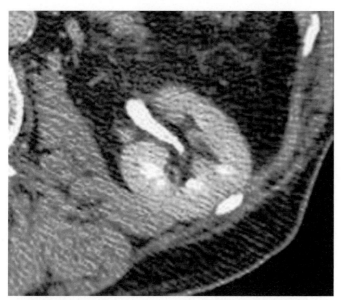

Figure 11.1   A

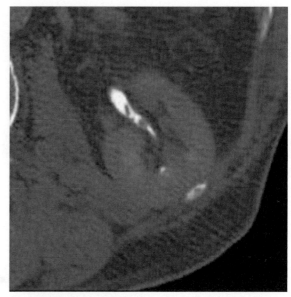

Figure 11.1   B

Findings: Axial excretory phase image (A), viewed utilizing standard soft tissue windowing, demonstrates a nondistended left renal collecting system. No masses are identified and there is no urothelial wall thickening. In comparison, when the same image is assessed with wider windows (B), three distinct filling defects, each measuring 5 mm or less, can be identified.

Diagnosis: Multifocal transitional cell carcinoma

Potential Pitfall: Urinary tract pathology will be missed if images are reviewed using only standard soft tissue windowing.

Discussion: Due to volume averaging with high-attenuation excreted contrast material, some intrarenal collecting system,

ureteral, and bladder abnormalities will not be detectable if images are reviewed using only standard soft tissue windowing. This problem is more likely when the pathology is small or subtle, as in this case. In order to avoid this pitfall, it is essential that excretory phase images be reviewed utilizing wide windows (often set between 2,000 and 4,000 HU). In this patient, if the left intrarenal collecting system were viewed only with standard soft tissue windowing, it would have been interpreted erroneously as normal. Each of the tiny filling defects was subsequently determined to be a focus of transitional cell carcinoma (see Cases 10-4 and 10-5).

History: 47-year-old male with recurrent obstructing ureteral calculi and urinary tract infection.

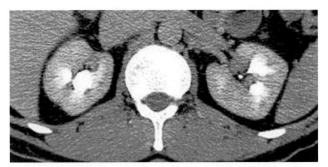

Figure 11.2   A

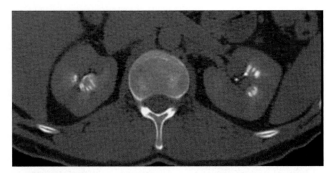

Figure 11.2   B

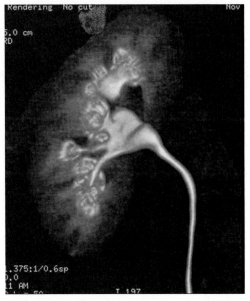

Figure 11.2   C

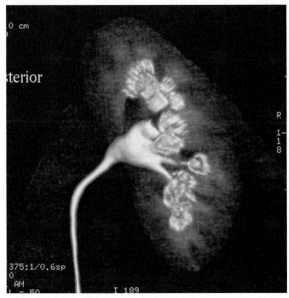

Figure 11.2   D

Findings: Excretory phase axial image from a CT urogram (A), viewed at soft tissue windows, demonstrates prominent calices bilaterally. Some of the visualized centrally located high-attenuation contrast material may actually reside in the renal pyramids; however, when using soft tissue windows the appearance is most consistent with a prominent papillary blush. In comparison, when the same image is viewed with wide windows (B), discrete linear rays of contrast-enhanced urine are identified in the renal pyramids. Similar findings are demonstrated in both kidneys on the volume-rendered images (C, D).

Diagnosis: Renal tubular ectasia

Potential Pitfall: Urinary tract pathology will be missed if images are reviewed using only standard soft tissue windowing.

Discussion: Occasional intrarenal collecting system, ureteral, and bladder abnormalities will not be detectable if images are reviewed using only standard soft tissue windowing. This problem is more likely when the pathology is small or subtle, as in this case. In order to avoid this pitfall, it is essential that excretory phase images be reviewed utilizing wide windows. In this patient, the discrete linear collections of opacified urine are identified only on images viewed with wide windows. The findings are diagnostic of renal tubular ectasia (see Cases 4-10 and 8-1).

History: 73-year-old male with intermittent microscopic hematuria.

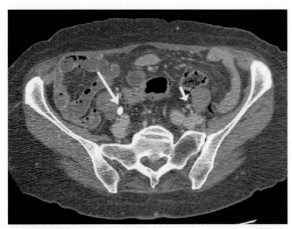

Figure 11.3   A

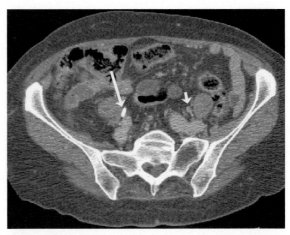

Figure 11.3   B

Findings: Two excretory phase axial images (A, B) demonstrate opacification of the right (long arrow) but not the left ureter (short arrow); however, both ureters can be seen to be normal in caliber.

Diagnosis: Left ureteral polyp

Potential Pitfall: Nonopacification of a nondilated ureter preventing detection of pathology.

Discussion: There are three reasons why urinary tract segments may not be opacified on CT urograms: (i) obstruction resulting in delayed excretion into usually dilated renal collecting systems and ureters; (ii) peristalsis in normal nondilated ureters; and (iii) layering of excreted contrast material in dilated portions of the renal collecting systems, ureters, and urinary bladder. Intrarenal collecting system and ureteral pathology is usually detectable when present in the dilated urinary tract. In particular, the cause of obstruction is frequently identified. In comparison, tiny abnormalities in unopacified nondistended portions of the intrarenal collecting systems and ureters may be impossible to detect, as in this case, in which a small left ureteral polyp was later diagnosed at the level illustrated here.

There are a number of possible approaches to the problem of unopacified nondilated urinary tract segments. Some radiologists obtain additional, more delayed, axial CT images, whereas others obtain delayed digital scout (or scan projection) radiographs. Still others perform no additional imaging and report these segments as normal, with the understanding that in rare instances, such as in the case illustrated here, abnormalities will be missed.

History: Elderly male with gross hematuria and negative cystoscopy.

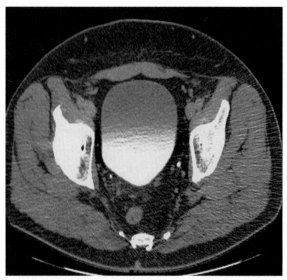

Figure 11.4 A

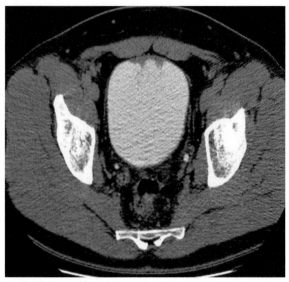

Figure 11.4 B

Findings: Excretory phase axial CT urography image obtained with the patient supine (A) demonstrates layering of opacified urine in the bladder. The bladder wall is not thickened and no intraluminal filling defects are identified. The second image (B), obtained several minutes later, after the patient was removed from the scanner and ambulated, shows that the contrast material and urine are now evenly mixed in the bladder. Irregular thickening along the anterior bladder wall is now apparent.

Diagnosis: Transitional cell carcinoma of the bladder

Potential Pitfall: Incomplete opacification of the bladder may prevent detection of bladder wall or luminal abnormalities.

Discussion: If the patient is kept in the supine position after contrast material excretion begins, urine containing contrast material will layer posteriorly in the bladder. Although many bladder lesions in the anterior aspect of the bladder can still be detected in this circumstance (outlined by lower water attenuation unopacified urine), this layering phenomenon may also result in failure to detect an occasional bladder lesion. This pitfall is particularly problematic in patients such as this, who can have normal cystoscopy. Indeed, the two blind spots during flexible cystoscopy are along the anterior wall of the bladder and at the bladder base. It is particularly important that these two areas be optimally imaged during CT urography. In order to do this, several measures may be taken to minimize the amount of unopacified urine in the bladder. Patients can be asked to void completely prior to CT urography. Alternatively, patients can be asked to roll over on the CT table several times and/or to ambulate just prior to excretory phase image acquisition. Others are willing to accept a slight decrease in study sensitivity. Without these maneuvers, CT urography technique is more straightforward and more simply performed because the patient can remain stationary. (Case courtesy of Nigel C. Cowan, Oxford University, Oxford, UK.)

CASE 11-5

History: 75-year-old female with hematuria.

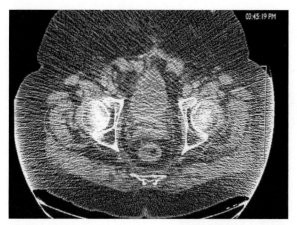

Figure 11.5   A

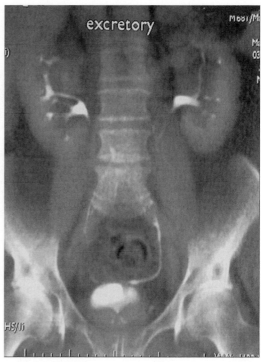

Figure 11.5   B

Findings: Single excretory phase axial image (A) has been obtained prior to excretion of injected contrast material into the bladder. The bladder contour is lobulated; however, the bladder wall is not markedly thickened. Average intensity projection image (B) demonstrates apparent wall thickening at the bladder base. Both images have a "grainy" appearance. A coronal excretory phase average intensity projection image obtained several minutes later demonstrates a small amount of contrast material in the bladder.

Diagnosis: Transitional cell carcinoma

Potential Pitfall: Reduced signal-to-noise ratio in large patients limits evaluation of the bladder.

Discussion: This patient is large. The increased soft tissue produces more x-ray beam scatter and there is a reduced signal-to-noise ratio. Generated axial images appear grainy and are of limited quality. This likely contributed to the inability to detect an 8-cm bladder neoplasm, that was subsequently identified at cystoscopy, in this patient.

History: Elderly patient with gross hematuria.

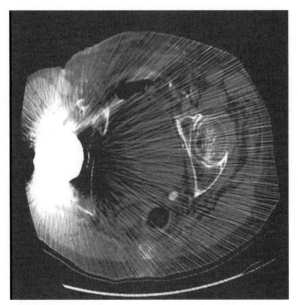

Figure 11.6

Findings: Excretory phase axial image demonstrates extensive artifact from a metallic right hip prosthesis. This limits visualization of nearly the entire pelvis, but particularly the right side of the bladder.

Diagnosis: Transitional cell carcinoma

Potential Pitfall: Metallic structures, such as hip prostheses, create extensive artifact and may prevent detection of urinary tract abnormalities.

Discussion: Hip prostheses result in extensive artifact and severely limit assessment of the bladder. In this case, a bladder cancer is present on the right but cannot be detected due to prosthesis artifact. Fortunately, follow-up cystoscopy was performed and demonstrated the neoplasm. (Case courtesy of Nigel C. Cowan, MD, FRCP, FRCR, Oxford University, Oxford, UK.)

History: Middle-aged female with persistent microscopic hematuria.

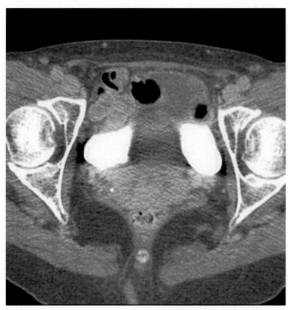

Figure 11.7 A

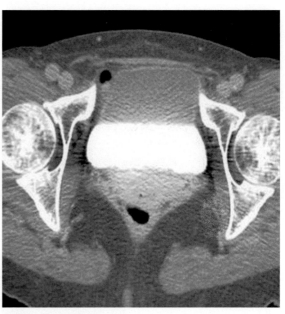

Figure 11.7 B

Findings: Two excretory phase axial images of the bladder illustrated using soft tissue windowing (A–B), obtained with the patient supine, demonstrate the bladder to be normal in size and shape. The bladder wall is not thickened and no filling defects/masses are identified in the unopacified or opacified portions of the bladder. (This was also the case when these images were viewed at wide windows.) The posterior impression on the cephalad image (A) represents volume average with the anteverted uterine fundus.

Diagnosis: Carcinoma in situ of the bladder

Potential Pitfall: Some urinary tract neoplasms will not be detectable even when the adjacent portions of the urinary tract are well opacified.

Discussion: This patient was subsequently referred for cystoscopy, at which time irregularity of the mucosa was noted along the right posterior aspect of the bladder wall, caudal to the right ureterovesical junction. A biopsy revealed carcinoma in situ.

Although CT urography is more sensitive in detecting urinary tract neoplasms than excretory urography or cystography, it does not detect all tumors. Microscopic tumor foci and carcinoma in situ in particular may be undetectable, even when the urinary tract is opacified optimally. In this instance, the bladder lumen adjacent to the wall containing the carcinoma in situ was well-opacified and the bladder wall visualized. Despite this, the neoplasm was not detectable, even in retrospect.

History: 52-year-old male with one episode of gross hematuria.

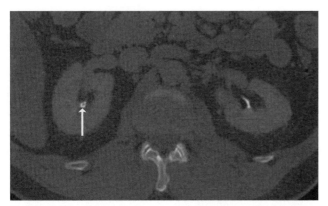

Figure 11.8 A

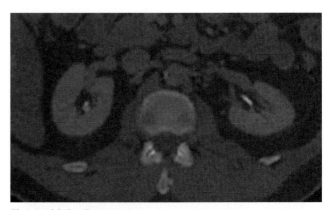

Figure 11.8 B

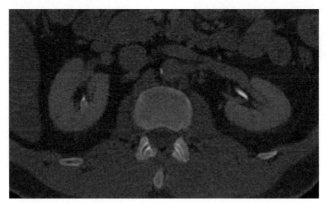

Figure 11.8 C

Findings: Excretory phase axial images obtained through the midportions of each kidney (A) demonstrate a small soft tissue attenuation filling defect (arrow) in a right renal calyx. On contiguous, more caudal images (B, C), this can be seen to merely represent a pronounced impression by a renal papilla.

Diagnosis: Prominent normal renal papilla

Potential Pitfall: Prominent renal papillae can mimic small intrarenal collecting system filling defects and can be mistaken for small urothelial tumors.

Discussion: Although renal papillae are occasionally prominent and can be mistaken for intrarenal collecting system pathology, this is not usually a problem, as long as the radiologist is aware that the pyramids can have a variable appearance and can invaginate fairly deeply into the calices, creating a convex caliceal shape (see Case 4-3). It is often helpful to note that other papillae in the same patient have a similar appearance. This appearance is responsible for the normal caliceal cupping often seen during excretory urography (which is also seen on coronal reformatted and three-dimensional images obtained at CT urography).

CASE 11-9

History: 77-year-old female with recurrent gross hematuria.

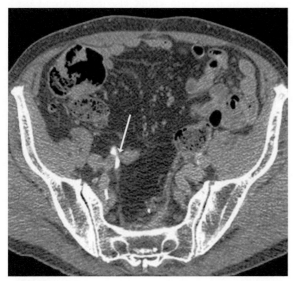

Figure 11.9   A

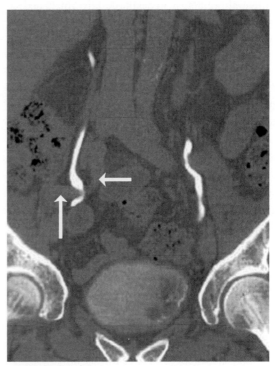

Figure 11.9   B

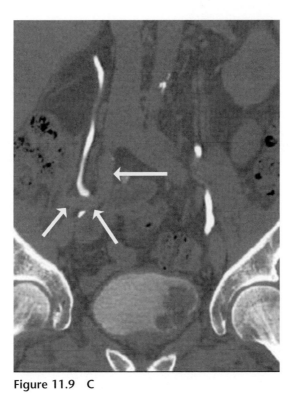

Figure 11.9   C

Findings: Axial excretory phase image (A) demonstrates a focal area of mid to distal right ureteral narrowing (arrow). The ureteral wall also appears slightly thickened in this region. This area is also displayed on two contiguous thin section coronal images (B, C), on which the right ureteral deviation can be seen to be due to a prominent right common iliac vein (arrows). The coronal images also demonstrate a large lobulated mass in the left side of the bladder.

Diagnosis: Crossing vessels

Potential Pitfall: Crossing arteries and veins may cause intrarenal collecting system or ureteral narrowing and may be mistaken for small filling defects or focally thickened urothelium.

Discussion: In this patient, the gross hematuria is explained by the large bladder cancer. The cause of the right ureteral narrowing is also seen on the coronal images but more difficult to identify on the axial image. However, the prominent right common iliac vein would also be apparent on axial images if the entire data set were reviewed sequentially at a workstation.

Arteries and veins can produce prominent impressions on the intrarenal collecting system and ureters, which can be mistaken for filling defects. This phenomenon has long been known to occur on excretory urography, typically affecting the upper pole renal infundibula; however, renal pelvic and ureteral impressions can also occur. These impressions are typically linear, although the linear morphology is often more difficult to appreciate on axial CT images. Also, the vessels themselves are often identified during CT urography.

CASE 11-10

History: Patient with known pelvic kidney and multiple urinary tract infections.

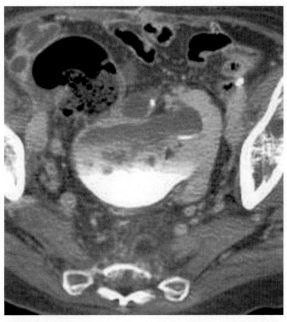

Figure 11.10

Findings: Axial excretory phase image demonstrates layering of excreted contrast material in the dilated pelvis of a left-sided pelvic kidney. Multiple irregularly shaped filling defects are noted in the middle of the renal pelvis at the same level as the interface between the opacified and unopacified urine.

Diagnosis: Mucus in a pelvic kidney

Potential Pitfall: Many different types of filling defects (blood clots, fungus balls, sloughed papillae, mucus, and occasional pedunculated neoplasms) may resemble one another.

Discussion: When CT urography includes unenhanced CT images, nearly all urinary tract calculi will be demonstrated;

however, other types of filling defects may have a similar appearance. Urothelial neoplasms are often distinguishable by their mucosal origin and contrast enhancement. Occasionally, acute or subacute blood clots will be recognized by their high attenuation on unenhanced images (ranging up to 60 to 80 HU); however, over time their attenuation will decrease. Finally, fungus balls and sloughed papillae may also have soft tissue attenuation.

Another rare cause of filling defects is mucus. Mucus, which can be seen when the urinary tract is anastomosed to bowel or merely due to urinary tract irritation/inflammation, is of little or no consequence.

History: 64-year-old with gross hematuria following ileal loop urinary diversion.

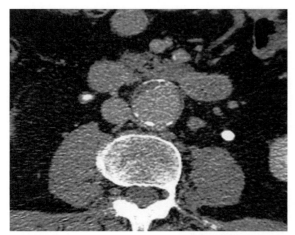

Figure 11.11   A

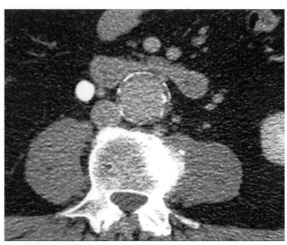

Figure 11.11   B

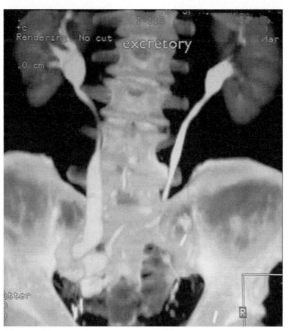

Figure 11.11   C

Findings: Two excretory phase axial images are provided. The first (A) demonstrates that both ureters are well-opacified. There is no filling defect bilaterally and the left ureteral wall is not thickened. In contrast, a thin circumferential rim of soft tissue attenuation surrounds the right ureter. On an excretory phase axial image obtained 2.5 minutes later (B), the left ureter is no longer opacified. The right ureter is more distended, and its wall is no longer thickened. The volume-rendered coronal image (C) demonstrates slight dilatation of both ureters with the exception of the proximal right ureter, which is smoothly narrowed.

Diagnosis: Normal right ureter

Potential Pitfall: Ureteral peristalsis may occasionally produce ureteral wall thickening.

Discussion: This case demonstrates that ureteral peristalsis can produce an abnormal appearance of the ureteral wall that mimics true pathologic thickening. Three-dimensional reconstructions cannot be used to detect urothelial wall thickening because these images do not delineate the urothelium; instead, they depict only the urinary tract lumen that it surrounds.

CASE 11-12

History: 32-year-old male with one episode of hematuria.

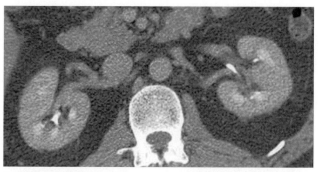

Figure 11.12 A

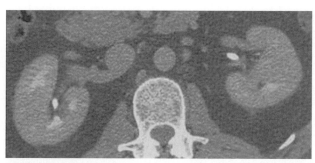

Figure 11.12 B

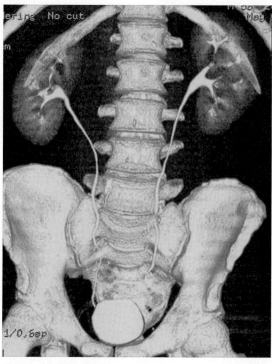

Figure 11.12 C

Findings: Axial excretory phase images filmed utilizing wide windowing (A, B) demonstrate increased attenuation in the renal pyramids. No discrete linear collections of contrast material are noted in these regions, however. The same finding is identified on the volume-rendered image (C).

Diagnosis: Normal renal papillary blush

Potential Pitfall: Prominent renal papillary blush can be mistaken for renal tubular ectasia.

Discussion: As with excretory urography, excretory phase CT urography images may demonstrate a dense renal papillary blush in some patients. This is a normal finding and can be distinguished from renal tubular ectasia on wide window images. With renal tubular ectasia, discrete linear rays of high attenuation are identified in the renal pyramids. When a prominent blush is present, the entire papillary region appears dense. When the CT urography images are viewed at standard soft tissue windows, prominent papillary blush and renal tubular ectasia usually have a similar appearance. The discrete linear collections of contrast material seen with renal tubular ectasia cannot be identified unless images are viewed at wide windows (see Case 11-2).

History: Elderly female with hematuria.

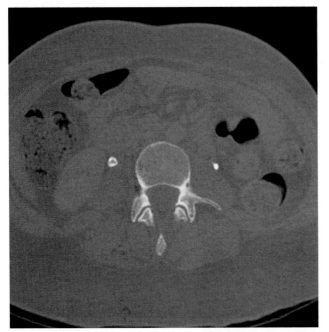

Figure 11.13   A

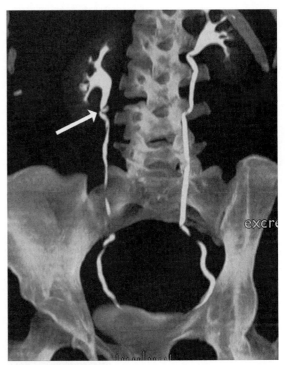

Figure 11.13   B

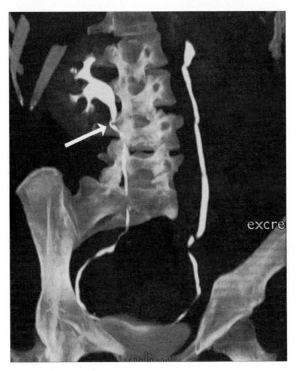

Figure 11.13   C

Findings: Excretory phase axial image (A), viewed with wide windows, reveals an apparent tiny filling defect within the proximal right ureter. The filling defect is not seen on bilateral oblique volume-rendered images (B, C). Instead, they demonstrate that the proximal right ureter is tortuous (arrows).

Diagnosis: Normal right ureter

Potential Pitfall: Ureteral tortuosity or "kinking" may create apparent ureteral filling defects on excretory phase axial CT urography images.

Discussion: Occasionally, ureters take a tortuous course. This phenomenon, which is more frequently encountered when patients are imaged during inspiration (since the diaphragm and, therefore, the kidneys are more caudally located), is also referred to as ureteral kinking. It is also more commonly seen in patients with ptotic kidneys and in patients who have had previous urinary tract obstruction. Ureteral kinking can cause apparent filling defects that can be mistaken for small urothelial neoplasms. These filling defects actually represent volume averaging of extra-ureteral tissue between two adjacent, but not immediately contiguous, segments of the ureter. The true nature of these apparent abnormalities is best appreciated when axial images are reviewed rapidly in succession at a workstation, where the tortuous and redundant course of the ureter will be readily apparent. Also, kinking may be identified on coronal or sagittal reformatted images and three-dimensional reconstructions.

History: 65-year-old patient who is status post cystectomy for bladder cancer.

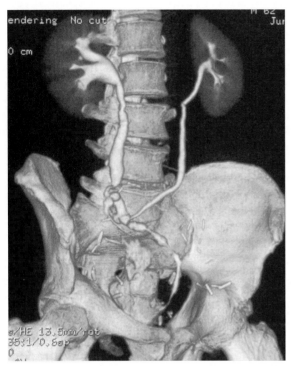

Figure 11.14   A

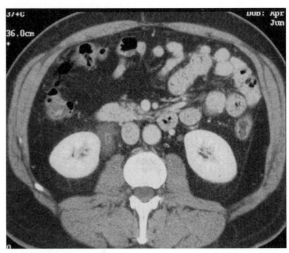

Figure 11.14   B

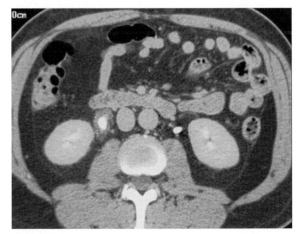

Figure 11.14   C

Findings: Volume-rendered three-dimensional image (A) demonstrates smooth narrowing of the right ureter and mild proximal intrarenal collecting system or renal pelvic dilatation. In contrast, nephrographic phase (B) and excretory phase (C) axial images demonstrate marked circumferential thickening surrounding the proximal right ureteral lumen. The lumen is not narrowed and does not have an irregular contour. On the nephrographic phase image (B), the urothelium can be seen as a thin enhancing rim surrounding the ureteral lumen, surrounded by extensive ureteral wall edema.

Diagnosis: Severe ureteritis

Potential Pitfall: Reliance on standard three-dimensional reconstructed images will result in underestimation of the severity of a detected abnormality.

Discussion: Circumferential thickening of a portion of the urinary tract often has little or no effect on the caliber or contour of the urinary tract lumen. For this reason, image reconstruction techniques that result primarily in visualization of the urinary tract lumen and not of the surrounding urothelium will fail to detect these abnormalities or, at least, will underestimate their severity. In this patient, it is possible that the slight smooth narrowing of the proximal right ureter might not have been identified had only the three-dimensional images been reviewed, particularly given the only mild dilatation of the right renal calices and right renal pelvis. Cases such as this serve to emphasize that source axial images or thin section reconstructed images (obtained using image thicknesses of no more than 2.5 to 5 mm) should always be reviewed.

CASE 11-15

History: 55-year-old female with intermittent bilateral flank pain.

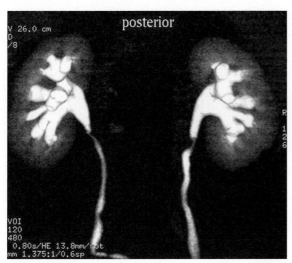

Figure 11.15 A

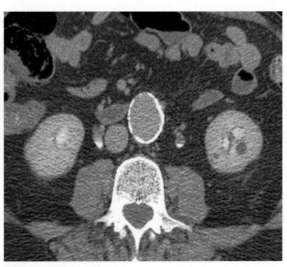

Figure 11.15 B

Findings: Posteroanterior excretory phase volume-rendered image (A) demonstrates mild to moderate bilateral pelvocaliectasis with pronounced smooth narrowing of both proximal ureters suggesting that bilateral ureteral strictures are present. On an excretory phase axial image (B), excreted contrast material can be identified layering dependently in both proximal ureters, which are actually mildly dilated rather than strictured.

Diagnosis: Mild bilateral proximal ureterectasis

Potential Pitfall: Layering of contrast-enhanced excreted urine can produce the appearance of urinary tract narrowing or other morphologic abnormality on three-dimensional reconstructed images.

Discussion: Excreted contrast material typically layers dependently in dilated portions of the urinary tract. This almost always occurs within the bladder (which is the largest urinary reservoir), although layering can also be seen in renal pelves, intrarenal collecting systems, and ureters when these segments are distended. In this patient, both ureters are dilated. Excreted contrast-enhanced urine has layered in both proximal ureters posterior to unopacified urine. Due to the shape of the ureters, the layered contrast material has created the appearance of strictures in the proximal ureters. This problem can be identified if the axial excretory phase images are reviewed.

Layering of excreted contrast material in dilated portions of the urinary tract can be prevented if the patient is moved fairly vigorously after contrast material injection but prior to excretory phase image acquisition. This can be done by asking the patient to ambulate between acquisitions and by having the patient turn from the supine to the prone position and back when he or she is returned to the scanner.

History: 65-year-old patient with gross hematuria.

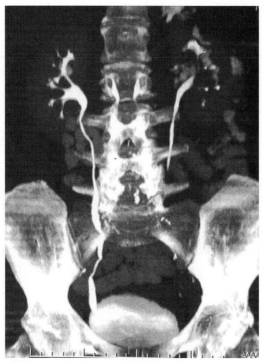

Figure 11.16

Findings: Volume-rendered image demonstrates nondilated intrarenal collecting systems and ureters bilaterally, although the distal half of the left ureter is not seen. The bladder is normal in caliber. Amorphous high-attenuation material is noted adjacent to the left intrarenal collecting system but also in the mid abdomen and upper pelvis.

Diagnosis: Oral contrast material imaged during CT urography

Potential Pitfall: Artifacts are created on three-dimensional reconstructed images when oral contrast material is inadvertently administered prior to CT urography.

Discussion: Oral contrast material should not be administered prior to CT urography if high-quality, three-dimensional, reconstructed images are to be obtained. Oral contrast material will be superimposed over portions of the urinary tract and limit their visualization on thick-slab reformatted images, such as the volume-rendered image in this case. As with many other potential pitfalls, the cause of these opacities can be identified on the axial images.

History: 57-year-old male with hematuria.

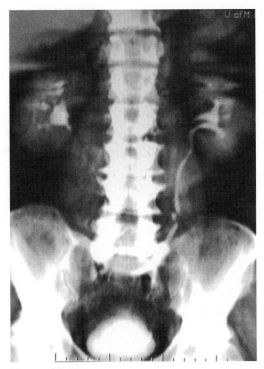

Figure 11.17

Findings: A single, average intensity, projection image demonstrates nondilated intrarenal collecting systems. Nearly the entire left ureter is opacified, as is the bladder; however, large portions of the right ureter are not seen. Extensive upper abdominal artifact creates large wedge-shaped areas of low attenuation that distort the appearance of both kidneys.

Diagnosis: Normal CT urogram

Potential Pitfall: Motion artifact limiting assessment of the urinary tract.

Discussion: Although multidetector CT scanners are extremely fast, artifact can still be created if the patient moves during the short time required for image acquisition. Portions of the urinary tract will not be clearly imaged and linear artifacts will be created on reformatted or three-dimensionally reconstructed images. There is no acceptable solution to this problem, other than rescanning the patient once he or she is able to lie still.

History: 75-year-old woman status post previous cystectomy and creation of a neobladder.

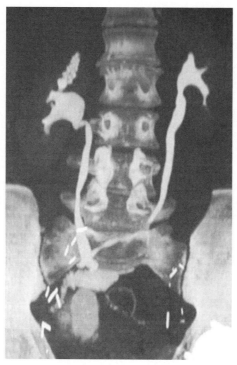

Figure 11.18

Findings: A volume-rendered image reveals an ovoid cluster of high-attenuation foci overlying the upper pole of the right kidney, immediately adjacent to the right upper pole calyx.

Diagnosis: Cholelithiasis

Potential Pitfall: Extra-urinary tract abdominal calcification overlying the kidneys can be mistaken for urinary tract calculi on three-dimensional reconstructed images.

Discussion: Occasionally, extra-urinary tract intra-abdominal calcifications can be confused with calcifications or stones in the urinary tract on three-dimensional reconstructed images. In this case, multiple gallstones overlie the upper pole of the right kidney. Based on the single provided image, the differential diagnosis would also include stones in a large right upper pole caliceal diverticulum or a dilated calyx. This case illustrates a problem that can occur if one relies exclusively on three-dimensional reconstructed images. Review of axial images (or of thin section reformatted images) usually identifies the source of any adjacent high-attenuation foci.

SUGGESTED READINGS

1. Caoili EM, Cohan RH, Korobkin M, et al. Urinary tract abnormalities: initial experience with multi-detector row CT urography. *Radiology*. 2002;222:353–360.

2. Caoili EM, Inampudi P, Cohan RH, et al. Multidetector CT urography of upper tract urothelial neoplasms. *Am J Roentgenol*. 2005;184: 1973–1881.

3. Noroozian M, Cohan RH, Caoili EM, et al. Multislice CT urography: state of the art. *Br J Radiol*. 2004;77:S74–S86.

INDEX

Figures are indicated by page numbers followed by *f*. Tables are indicated by page numbers followed by *t*.

partially opacified obstructed, 15
unopacified obstructed, 15
Urolithiasis, extracorporeal shock wave
    lithotripsy for, 51, 51*f*
Uroselectan, 2
Urothelial wall, thickening of, 185–186, 185*f*
UTI. *See* Urinary tract infection

V

Vascular malformation, partially thrombosed,
    renal sinus, 137–138*f*, 138
Vesicoureteric reflux (VUR), 145
Vesicovaginal fistula, 250, 250*f*
Vessels, crossing, 261*f*, 262
Voiding dysfunction, 44–45*f*
Volume-rendered image
    of acute infectious ureteritis, 91, 91*f*
    of acute pyelonephritis, 56, 56*f*
    of benign prostatic hyperplasia, 231, 231*f*
    of bladder calculi with pyelitis, 52–53, 52*f*
    of bladder cancer, 37, 37*f*, 70*f*, 71,
        236*f*, 237
    of bladder diverticulum, 229*f*, 230
    of branched calculus, with hydrocalyx,
        155, 155*f*
    of cake kidney, 68, 68*f*
    of calculi with pyelitis, 52–53, 52*f*
    of collecting system, duplication of, 36, 36*f*,
        44–45*f*, 146*f*, 147
    of compound calyx, 33, 33*f*
    computed tomography urography, 29*f*, 30

of congenital calyceal diverticulum,
    148–149, 148*f*
of Crohn disease,
    corticomedullary phase, 72, 72*f*
    nephrographic phase, 72, 72*f*
of cross fused renal ectopia, 156, 156*f*
of duplication collecting system, 36, 36*f*
of flank pain, 74–75, 74*f*, 76–77*f*, 77
of forniceal rupture, 57–58, 57*f*
of hematuria, 29*f*, 30, 33, 33*f*, 36, 36*f*,
    52–53, 52*f*, 65*f*, 66, 104, 104*f*
of horseshoe kidney, 39, 39*f*, 157, 157*f*
of ileal neobladder, 236*f*, 237, 238*f*, 239
of kidney with calculi, 67, 67*f*
of leiomyoma, 227*f*, 228
of low back pain,, arterial phase, 67, 67*f*
of lymphomatous mass, 197–198, 197*f*
of medullary sponge kidney, 143, 143*f*
of mild bilateral proximal ureterectasis,
    269, 269*f*
of narrowed ureter with atherosclerotic iliac
    artery, 34*f*, 35
of nephrogenic adenoma, 193–194*f*, 194
of nephrolithiasis, 68–69, 68*f*, 86, 86*f*
of nonobstructive calculi, 57–58, 57*f*,
    65–66, 65*f*
of normal papillary blush, 265, 265*f*
of normal ureter, 264, 264*f*
of obstructing ureteral calculus, 57–58, 57*f*,
    70*f*, 71
of orthotopic ureterocele, 232*f*, 233
of parapelvic cyst, 104, 104*f*

of post-radiofrequency ablation of collecting
    system, 160*f*, 161
of ptotic kidney, 37, 37*f*
of reflux nephropathy, 144*f*, 145
of renal abscess, 86, 86*f*
of renal calculi, 56, 56*f*
of renal cell carcinoma, 160*f*, 161
of renal fusion anomaly, 157, 157*f*
of renal insufficiency, 47*f*, 48
of renal pelvis calculi with hydronephrosis,
    51, 51*f*
of renal tubular acidosis, 76–77*f*, 77
of renal tubular ectasia, 254, 254*f*
of retroperitoneal sarcoma, 154, 154*f*
of retroperitoneal sarcoma, 154, 154*f*
of segmental multicystic dysplasia,
    139–140*f*, 140
of severe ureteritis, 268, 268*f*
of transitional cell carcinoma, 163*f*, 164,
    166, 166*f*, 173*f*, 174, 175, 175*f*, 212*f*,
    213, 215–216*f*, 216, 219–220, 219*f*,
    221, 221*f*
of ureteral duplication, 146*f*, 147
of urinary tract infection, 56, 56*f*,
    76–77*f*, 77
of urolithiasis, 51, 51*f*
VUR. *See* Vesicoureteric reflux

X

Xanthogranulomatous pyelonephritis,
    3, 74–75, 74*f*, 94, 94*f*, 169*f*, 170